MEMOIRS OF A
MIDWIFE IN HUNGARY

1928-1956

Mária Szécsi

Solutions LaniSys Inc.

In my eyes I still shed heated tears,
as my past memories I summon,
since tears and blood are cost of deliveries,
and of all novelties, as known by each woman!

ZSENI VÁRNAI: IN MILLIONS' HEARTS

CONTENTS

GRANDSON'S PROLOGUE

Dear Reader,

Let me bring this book, originally intended for a Hungarian readership, closer to your use with some supplementary comments on the occasion of its electronic English publication.

The stories described in the book took place between 1928 and 1956 in the most impoverished rural districts of Hungary. These stories were also told to me by my grandmother when I was a child. As for me, who spent most of my winter and summer childhood vacations with her in the little village of Orosháza in south-eastern Hungary, these stories still come to life in my imagination. Originally, it was not the storyline that grabbed my attention but rather the sense of experience and security that resonated in it. My grandmother, though having worked only in a tiny field of medicine, gained so much confidence in preserving human well-being through her decades-long struggle of performed deliveries that no matter what my health problem was she could always deal with it perfectly on her own. Sometimes we didn't even share these 'natural medicinal treatments' with my mother who, though she worked as a volunteer-nurse during World War II, didn't have extensive knowledge in this type of healing, and I presume she didn't have the necessary confidence to use them.

My grandmother had to develop techniques due to the daily constraint and scarcity of resources. The example of giving a patient suffering from fluid-loss and drying-out one spoon of cold milk every hour exhibits this nicely. In the absence of infusion and other tools and with the lack of hospital conditions, my grandmother could still ensure the normalization of a patient's fluid level and bring him out of a critical condition.

For me, the stories found in the book are "natural" in the sense that I do not find anything surreal in the behavior of its characters, because these behaviors were accepted and everyday norms of rural society. The fact that taking care of household animals often had higher priority even for childbearing women than childbearing itself, or the fact that men often gave minimal help in these deliveries, does not classify the character of these people but rather sheds light on norms accepted by everyone in those societies.

As long as we want to draw valid conclusions from a given age, we have to acquaint ourselves in depth with the everyday life, habits and routines of this age in the fashion experienced by its people. Such works, showing everyday life itself, can bring the given age closer to the reader than a historical, political or economic explanation.

The dictation, documentation and later electronic publication of this book serve this very purpose of bringing the age of our great-grandparents closer to the reader.

Getting back to the book, my grandmother was born in 1900 in Transylvania, which was then part of Hungary. Along with her sisters, she moved to the Hungarian plain and married at the age of twenty a bootmaker near the village of Orosháza. She had her first daughter, my mother, at twenty-two. She attended to the chores around the house, and her husband earned credit in the area as a diligent tradesman. Nonetheless, her husband, who was fit as a fiddle all his life, died abruptly to the shock of all when she was twenty-seven. My grandmother who had neither a trade nor wealth on which to get by was left alone with her five-year-old daughter. Their future turned uncertain in an instant.

Then, she heard that they were about to start a boarding-school, one-year obstetrical program at the University of Szeged. The graduates were promised a certificate with which they could start a private practice. She could not take her five-year-old daughter with her to the institution, so she asked her own mother to come from Transylvania and take care of the daughter for a year. My mother later told me her experience about visiting my grandmother at this institution. As they had no money, they had to make the sixty-kilometer journey on foot. They had to return the next day because this institution originally did not allow family stays; that being the case, my grandmother still did manage to put them up secretly on the premises at least for one night.

I don't know how this midwifery profession came to her mind but eventually it became her trademark. She became the "midwife" or simply the familiar "Miss Mária" in her district. She worked for around thirty years as a professional private midwife. It is hard to give an exact number of her performed deliveries. Her own documented, handwritten records, which she entered after every delivery, give 1369 deliveries. Given the fact that some records are entirely missing for certain years of her activity and that she no longer documented her activity in the 1950s when she was working for an obstetrical clinic, the actual number of all her performed deliveries must be much higher, perhaps even twice this number. In the year of 1941 alone, she performed 299 deliveries in the often primitive conditions well-described in the book. When she was called for, she usually reached the place on foot or by bicycle, be it three in the morning or eleven in the evening.

As she wrote it in her memoirs: "I never felt afraid; my only concern was to arrive in time!" She knew she was needed and counted upon.

According to her kept records, throughout her career she lived in twelve different settlements, mainly in Békés county, which was an impoverished, overwhelmingly rural region at the time, but also in other parts of Hungary.

She retired at fifty-six but kept saying even at seventy that she felt enough energy to continue to work at the clinic should it be necessary. After her retirement she married again, to a widowed husband whose former wife's delivery had been performed by her. Uncle Gyuri, my grandmother's new husband, became my new grandfather whom I came to admire a great deal. They lived in Orosháza, the village where my grandmother used to work a great deal during her career.

When I spent my childhood years with her at the village, it was only natural that wherever we went, my grandmother was always recognized and greeted by someone who, in turn, started retelling the lives of their children who had been delivered by my grandmother.

I can still remember the occasion when we were spending time at the village's public pool and a lady with her adult son came up to us. This son happened to be the rather strict lifeguard of the pool. He, who had almost military command over the whole area with a beep of his whistle, now sat down to talk to us in a deeply touched, almost adolescent manner. This made me realize how much people can be moved by a previous act of kindness. Even if they can express gratitude only later on, this thankfulness stays within them, and it is a great feeling to experience it.

My grandmother's chosen profession and her experience throughout her career had a huge impact not only on her daughter but also on me. Although I did not become involved in any medical profession, I still tried to remain in the vicinity of the field of medicine and health care. As an engineer, I became specialized in the development of medical equipment, conducted physiological experiments and tried to describe and comprehend the work of the respiratory system in the language of mathematics.

I trust that my grandmother's memoirs will serve as an exciting experience to the reader. I also hope that this book's atmosphere will exhibit more fully a world where independent and decisive action was needed, regardless of the circumstances or the available resources.

Her grandson – Zsolt Balassy

Budapest, August, 2020

MIDWIFE OR OBSTETRICIAN?

The idea to become a midwife would probably have never occurred to me had it not been for the death of my husband. He passed away on March 15, 1927, leaving me alone with my five-year-old daughter and without a breadwinner in the family. What money my husband had previously earned, we could modestly get by on, although we could not put any aside.

In the village where we lived, there was an old midwife with whom I talked a lot. She told me how much she loved her profession, shared her experiences about child bearings and deliveries and talked about the connections she had developed with the pregnant mothers during her career. Even though the thought to apply to a midwifery course started to appeal to me more and more, I knew I had no money to pay the tuition.

I was ready to take any job I could find to save some money for my education; I was a reaper on a grain field, I took part in silkworm breeding, I fattened pigs, and in the meantime I tried to get prepared for the midwifery admission test.

The test took place in 1927 in the city of Szeged.[1] Out of the 80 applicants, 45 were admitted, myself included. We were told that the course would start on September 1, 1927, and that we should show up on that date at 9 Fodor Street in Szeged. They explained that the course would last for 10 months and we had to pay the accommodation, tuition, and exam fees ourselves. Moreover, we had to bring our own bedclothes and school uniform, clean the wards in the morning, deliver food to the patients and care for them as needed. Classes took place in the afternoon, and we could study for them in the evening. I was so happy I got admitted that I felt I could power through anything at the moment. I hurried home so that I could save enough money for my course starting in September.

In the beginning, studying was hard, but I always prepared for my classes diligently. I had great oral exam results and I passed the final examination with flying colors.

We received a 10-month training in school, which included a theoretical as well as a practical component. Evidently, this short period of time only enabled us to acquire a basic knowledge of anatomy. They did not even teach us how to give an injection to a patient, because, at that time, only doctors were allowed to do so. However, later on in our careers, we would have needed this skill, as doctors were not always present.

Life did, without a doubt, teach us how to be autonomous, ingenious and tenacious in our profession.

With my obtained degree, I went home happy. As a state-commissioned obstetrician had already been working in the village, I could only start a private practice. I was allowed to ask up to 12 pengős[2] after each delivery, which the local families could rarely afford. These families instead called the commissioned obstetrician who was bound to administer each childbirth free of charge. Therefore, I could hardly get by and had to sell clothes and bed linen so that I could buy food for myself.

Finally, in 1929, it came to my attention that in a neighboring village a midwife position was advertised. I handed in my application to the assistant notary at the local village office. He told me that the name of the successful applicant would be announced in the newspaper.

Because a local midwife's contract meant 50 pengős a month, which would have given me a living wage, I desperately wanted to get the position. I was looking forward to the results in the local newspaper, but found out to my great astonishment that they decided to choose an applicant from a distant region because, according to them, nobody from any nearby village had applied for the position.

The next day, I went to see the chief notary to ask him what had happened to my application. He immediately questioned his assistant, who claimed to have accidentally left mine in his drawer. I can't recall the details, but the assistant—since it wasn't his first time being careless—was seriously rebuked and was ordered to pay me 50 pengős every month until a new position was posted. Eventually, he visited me at my place after the incident and explained to me that he had a family, no means to pay the amount, and asked me to be so kind as not to claim the money. Although I had serious financial difficulties, I advised him to be less careless next time and told him that it was not necessary for him to pay me.

A new position was posted later on, for which I successfully applied. On the basis of my documents, they unanimously asked me to be the midwife of the community.

The designated community also included a large farm district. My responsibilities consisted of conducting deliveries free of charge—as I got paid by the village—, checking on the mothers and bathing their babies for eight days following their deliveries.

In those days, the poor were numerous and gave birth to children continually. Even though I still had my license for private practice, there were so many poor childbearing mothers that I had time only to pursue my community practice, which yielded less income. Thus it took me many years until I could finally afford a bicycle, which was of great use in this profession.

I performed thousands of deliveries over my 28-year-long practice. In this book I would like to recount the most memorable cases that will serve as true depictions of the times when midwives like me had to strive in often primitive conditions to save lives.

In 1920s' Hungary, hospitals and obstetrical clinics existed only in towns. In the countryside there was only one doctor assigned to each village at best. If we needed the help of a doctor for a complicated delivery on a farm, we had to send for the one assigned to our district. Telephones and cars being rare in those times, a horse-drawn carriage was used for transportation, if there was one available at all. If a carriage was not available, which was the case most of the time, a person had to go on foot to inform the doctor. In this case, every single minute counted and the person undertaking the journey had to walk for long hours so that the midwife's call for assistance might reach the doctor. If the doctor was not visiting a patient and happened to be at home, he tried to come using any means of transportation available: on foot, by carriage, on horseback, or sometimes even by bicycle. If he managed to reach us, we at least had the presence of a doctor. Even though he was usually not an obstetrician by specialization, he was still a medical expert, which meant a great relief to us. When there was no doctor present—being a rather common case —the life of the mother or the newborn depended on the skill and ingenuity of the midwife and, honestly, on a bit of luck.

I was a community midwife for 25 years, after which I went on to work at an obstetrical clinic for 3 years, which makes up 28 years of practice in total. How many thrills and how much suffering and joy it was! It was such a good feeling that whenever I travelled, many out of the thousands of mothers still recognized me and cried out, "Miss Mária! How come you are here? Don't you recognize me?" And they started to recall the most memorable moments of their childbearing.

I loved my profession. It was always my dream to see my daughter follow me on the same path, knowing all the experience I could have shared with her. Unfortunately, this dream did not come true —a medical career did not appeal to her. "Maybe my grandchild will follow!" I kept telling myself. He happened to be a boy; and even though he couldn't be a midwife, he still could have embarked on a medical career. Alas, he chose a different path too.

BARGAINING
FOR A COW

Saving lives on rural farms often depended on the resourcefulness and skill of midwives.

On one occasion, as I was preparing to go to bed, somebody knocked on my window. Outside, I saw a man in his forties standing on the street with a carriage behind him.

"Miss Mária!" he shouted. "Please check on my wife; she needs help! She doesn't feel well. As you know she is expecting a baby, but the date of expected delivery is supposed to be two weeks from now."

I quickly got dressed, took the two midwife bags that were always prepared for emergencies, and was ready to go. I was about to get into the carriage when the man stopped me.

"I am sorry, but I urgently have to go to the next village. Please be so kind and go to see my wife on foot."

"Where do you live?" I asked him suspiciously.

"Here on farm Z," and he pointed a finger to a distance somewhere in the darkness.

"But that's a good way from here!" I exclaimed, but hardly had I looked around when he had whipped his horses and left as if his job was done here. He probably believed his conscience was clear since he had called the local midwife and his wife would not be alone after all.

I knew I had no time to waste, as every second could make the difference between life and death for the baby. I left alone on foot.

It was late at night when I arrived on farm Z. The wife was home with an eight-year-old boy. I examined her and concluded that the time of delivery had indeed arrived. Although everything seemed to be in order, I was still worried that I couldn't find a single person who could help me in case anything happened.

I kept asking the woman, "What was so urgent that made your husband leave your side and make me come here on foot? And anyway, how could you let your husband, who knew these were labor pains, leave you?" I had a hard time finding out that the husband's urgent business was a cow on sale at a bargain price. I knew that if any complications arose, we would be helpless. However, I did not mean to scare my patient by repeating that this abrupt leave was careless on her husband's part. I couldn't wait to finish the delivery.

As it was late at night, I sent the young boy to the kitchen to find himself a place to sleep because it was not his place to stay in the room of delivery. He obeyed me without a word. Clearly, he was so tired he could barely keep his eyes open.

The pains that preceded the labor gradually started to intensify, and by midnight the woman gave birth to a nice, blonde, chubby baby girl. After the delivery, however, the expulsion of the placenta took place far too slowly.

I examined her thoroughly and saw that some parts of the organ had not been expelled, which caused the mother to start bleeding.

In this case—as we had been taught cautiously in school—a doctor had to be sent for immediately. Unsurprisingly, they did not teach us what to do when we were alone in the middle of the night on a remote farm without a doctor nearby and without anyone who could be sent for one. The nearest inhabited place was a lung-sanatorium a couple of kilometers from the patient's home. "There must be a doctor there," I thought to myself. "But who should I send there? I cannot leave the patient here, therefore I cannot go myself." Because the poor woman's bleeding worsened, I didn't have much time to think. I entered the kitchen, hoping that the husband had come back, but, at first sight, I couldn't find anyone there. Then, all of a sudden, I noticed the boy in one corner, sleeping on two chairs that he put together. I found the idea of sending an eight-year old child absurd, but there was no alternative. When he slowly woke up, I addressed him.

"Young man, your mother is very sick and needs a doctor at once. Since your father is not at home, you have to go! You are a big, strong and brave boy and your help is essential right now. While you get dressed, I will write a letter that you must carry to the sanatorium. You will stay there until you find a doctor who is able to come here. It is dark and the sanatorium is far from here, but I am certain you will meet someone on your way whom you can ask to accompany you. Do not worry, you will most certainly find somebody!" I tried to encourage him.

He evidently understood what I said; without saying a word he put on his boots and coat and left with the letter.

The next hour was nerve-racking. I tried to use all my knowledge to reduce the bleeding.

At last, the boy appeared at the door with a doctor. Initially, the doctor entered the room irritated and said what a horrible idea it was for a midwife to call a lung-specialist to assist in a delivery. I told him that the sanatorium was the nearest inhabited place and the district doctor lived in the village, so it was impossible to send for him. I also explained to him that my patient was bleeding excessively and her husband, who was supposedly in the tavern by that time perhaps toasting the health of the newborn, had left her wife here so that he could buy a cow at a bargain price. The doctor, seeing that I had no other choice than to send the young boy for him to the sanatorium, concluded that I had solved the problem quite ingeniously indeed.

He gave the woman an injection that reduced the bleeding. In the meantime, they were preparing a carriage in the sanatorium to take her to a hospital.

About ten days after the incident, a carriage appeared in front of our house. The husband was taking his wife home from the hospital and they stopped by to thank me for my efforts. The man hid behind his wife's skirt when I told him that the purchase of his cow had almost cost his spouse's life.

A LETTER OF REPRIMAND

I was always afraid whenever I was asked to do a delivery at a remote, lonely farm. Sending for a doctor in those rural places in case of any complications was a great challenge. Our village didn't even have a local doctor, so I always had to send for one in the neighboring town. It is daunting to think how many difficult hours I had to suffer at these farms waiting for a doctor and using all my skills in order to save a newborn's life. Not to mention the fact that I was completely helpless in case a patient had to be taken to a hospital.

One evening, I was called to a delivery by a man. "We will take a horsecar[3] to my place instead of going on foot," he reassured me. As soon as he told me where he was taking me, I got anxious because I knew how far away this particular farm was. I knew I would not be able to send for a doctor there should it be necessary.

I told him that he should have brought his wife to the village by the horsecar. Had he done that, we could have taken his wife directly to the hospital to have her delivery. I said that by the time we get to the farm it would be late at night and we would be helpless in case we needed a doctor.

In the end, however, it was the husband who got angry. He demanded if I knew a way to take his wife to a hospital while not leaving the kids and the farm unattended for a long time. He also said that it was my duty as a local midwife to visit the mothers. Most importantly, he saw no reason to worry, as this would be the sixth delivery of his wife and everything should be fine. "All the previous five deliveries went well and a doctor's help was never required." To this he added, "Let's head out now, because my wife must be in severe pain by this time."

And thus, we left. Nonetheless, I could not calm myself down on the way, and I had this gut feeling that something would eventually go wrong. We walked to the rails and boarded the horsecar. The ride lasted for an hour until we finally reached the end of the rails. After the ride, we had to cross a forest on foot, beyond which I finally spotted the farm. It was already dark. The man led the way and I followed him stumbling on the deserted forest path.

When we finally arrived at the farm, the children had already been asleep and the pregnant mother was anxiously walking up and down in a room upstairs. I told her to stop moving and lie down somewhere since she must be in serious pain by this point. It even occurred to me that the time of delivery wasn't even close and perhaps her husband had only tried to frighten me with his comments. "Oh, I am in serious pain, but I never lie down until the very last moment," the wife told me. I kept an eye on the mother as I was washing my hands, but I didn't notice her being in pain at all.

I told her one more time to lie down so that I could examine her. "There's something wrong here," I thought to myself; but the woman did not let me examine her. She said she always lay down only at the last minute and nobody had examined her when she gave birth to her previous five children. After a long persuasion, I managed to make her lie down on the bed. No sooner had she done that than she cried out in agony and started to wail. I was not expecting anything like this, as she had borne all her pain without a word until that point. Previously, she managed to hide her pain so successfully that even I couldn't notice it. I asked her what happened, what she felt, what was wrong; but she was wailing so desperately that she couldn't even answer any of my questions.

We had learned during our midwifery course that a sudden, acute pain might appear in case of a uterine rupture, but I had never come across such a case in my career so far. I checked the heartbeat of both the fetus and the mother and they were all right.

I went to the kitchen and asked the man to fetch a carriage because his wife had to be taken to a hospital. I told him that a serious operation was most likely needed at this point.

The man did not seem to understand the gravity of the situation and answered that it was impossible to find a carriage until the sun came up. "Because sewing the wound is not an option for the mother, it doesn't matter how dark it is. Go to the nearest farm where they have a carriage and ask to borrow it! Be quick because every second could make the difference between life and death for the baby!" It took him quite some time to understand how serious the situation was, but finally he left and I was able to attend to the patient again.

It was already dark outside and it started raining so heavily that it caused boots to get stuck in the mud, making the journey a real challenge. The man also had some difficulty in waking up the owner of the next farm. The neighbor owned a carriage and horses but was unwilling to accompany him. When this poor man started to beg him and explained that his wife's life was on the line, the neighbor lent him the horses and the carriage that were kept in the barn. The owner, however, told him that he was so exhausted that he could not get up. After plowing all day, he strained his waist and was unable to move. The horses were exhausted too, in fact, but what was to be done when the problem was so grave.

Even though the man had never owned either a horse or a carriage in his life, he was excited as he went to the barn to harness the horses. As it was his first time doing this, he didn't know how to do it properly and placed the horses on the wrong sides in front of the carriage. He placed the horse that was used to walking on the right side of the carriage on the left side and the other one on the right side. He didn't understand why he couldn't make the horses pull the carriage and eventually ended up walking beside them. He had to lead them this way in order to make them move.

It took him a full hour to return to our farm with the carriage. I was glad when I heard its sound. We quickly put blankets and pillows in it to create a comfortable place for the woman. In the meantime, I was trying to figure out how we could get this heavy, pregnant woman into the carriage; she was in so much pain by this time that she was hardly able to move. Whenever I touched her, she started screaming.

At the beginning, her husband and I tried to lift her— unsuccessfully. As soon as we gave it a try, she tearfully begged us to leave her alone to die because she couldn't bear the pain of moving. This acute pain assured me of a prevailing uterine rupture, even if I had had my doubts about it before. I was thinking that some part of the fetus must have got stuck in the ruptured part of the uterus, hence tearing it further and causing terrible pain for the mother.

Following a quick break after our failed trials, I called back the husband, who had retreated to the kitchen in the meantime, and emphasized that we had no time to lose. "I know it will cause severe pain for your wife, but no matter how loudly she wails, we have to gently but firmly grab, lift and carry her outside to the carriage," I said to the husband. I had doubts about my physical strength, but I was confident that I would not drop his wife along the way.

I cannot describe the torment that the three of us had to go through until we finally managed to carry the mother to the carriage. Then, we had to face the next challenge; the man couldn't drive the horses properly because they were not put on the appropriate side at the front of the carriage. Of course, this was something he only realized after the incident. He had to get off the carriage again and lead the horses, walking beside them.

We took that long path across the dense forest once again, looking for the right direction while it was pitch dark. I sat next to the patient, checking her pulse and the heartbeat of the fetus. I still found both of them all right, which reassured me a bit. This is how we eventually reached the horsecar station, step-by-step.

Our torment continued here. We woke the driver up, waited till he got dressed and put the horses to the car. Then all together we lifted the poor woman and put her in the horsecar. This time it was the three of us who lifted the woman, which was certainly an easier task, at least for us. Notwithstanding this, the mother's pain was not relieved a bit. At last, we arrived at the village. Although there was no hospital here, there was at least a post office equipped with a telephone and therefore an ambulance could be called from the town. It was late at night, which meant that the office was closed. We had to go to the house of the postmaster, wait for him to come to the post office and then wait to get connected to a line on the telephone—a chain of nerve-racking events.

The ambulance quickly arrived and so we got promptly to town. In the obstetrical clinic, a young, novice lady was on duty at the time when we arrived there. I told her right away that we had brought a patient supposedly with a uterine rupture and that I wanted to speak to the doctor on duty. The lady, despite my request, asked me to keep a distance from her and leave the room, saying I was not disinfected. She said that the doctor would diagnose the patient and thus I could feel free to go home. Then, as I looked at myself, I realized that I wasn't disinfected indeed; my clothes had got wet and dirty partly from the rain and partly from the mud while we were trying to lift and place the patient from one car to the other. I didn't even make the impression of a medical employee, let alone a midwife.

I sent the husband back home so that his kids would not be alone. I took a seat in the corridor and waited, hoping to meet the doctor on duty. I waited for a long time, but nobody came to update me, so I knocked on the door and enquired whether the doctor made his diagnosis; after all, I was also interested in the results. The young nurse I talked to before came out of the room and explained that there was no uterine rupture at all, instead the placenta started to get expelled at an early stage. Nevertheless, I was adamant, having been with the patient and witnessed the symptoms first-hand, I declared that a uterine rupture was more probable in my opinion. The doctor on duty came out of the room to our loud debate and asked me to wait a bit for him to call the chief physician, who could examine the patient too. He arrived shortly, diagnosed the mother and ordered an operation to take place immediately. It seemed still possible to save the fetus, because the heartbeat was still satisfactory.

I waited until the end of the operation despite being exhausted. It was only in the morning that the chief doctor finally informed me that the fetus, unfortunately, did not make it through the operation, but the mother was all right. It was a uterine rupture indeed, as I suspected, but since the lower part of the uterus got torn and the head of the fetus got stuck there, the wound was sealed up and there was no internal bleeding.

I went home feeling broken and exhausted after the event. The thought that after all this torment and suffering we were not able to save the life of the fetus, only that of the mother, frustrated me.

I wanted to do one thing only at this point: go home to sleep and empty my mind of the day's events. Despite my wish, I noticed someone from a distance standing in front of the door of my house. As I got closer, a man hurried to me. "I am so glad you are here Miss Mária! My wife doesn't feel well and I think that her contractions have started. Please come with me! We live close by." And so I left again.

Two weeks had passed after the uterine rupture incident when the district doctor asked me to come to his office. He had received a disciplinary letter from the hospital, asking him to reprimand the local midwife for bringing in the patient too late to the hospital. I had been working with this doctor for a long time, and he was well aware of the nature of my job as well as that of the district where I worked. He was familiar with the situation on these remote farms too, where there was no neighboring farmer nearby who could offer help. He knew that the poor often did not have a horse or a carriage. He was also familiar with the often hopeless situation of a patient's transportation from these places. He didn't reprimand me at all, but instead showed me the letter and sighed wearily, "They should rather imagine how much better it would be for us as well to work in a well-equipped, clean hospital."

He then tore the letter to pieces and threw it in the trash.

THE MIDWIFE AND THE INTERNIST

Part I

In the 1920s it was extremely rare for a town or village to have a local doctor. I always had to send for one in the neighboring village whenever it was necessary for a delivery. When I heard that a young doctor was planning to settle in our village, I became very excited. Even though he was an internist and not an obstetrician, he still decided to reside in our village and I thought he could probably help us with deliveries if asked.

I soon had to ask for him, indeed, for a delivery in which the mother had a small perineal tear that had to be sewn up. On other occasions, I asked him to give injections. He always helped us readily, and thus it seemed that we would collaborate nicely in the future.

We had been working together for two years already when one night I was called to a delivery. I examined the woman and concluded that the fetus was lying in a transverse position. I could not hear the heartbeat of the fetus, which was worrisome, so I asked the mother when was the last time she felt her baby moving. "It's been more than a week by now," she said, so I suspected that it must have been a perinatal death. In the meantime, the patient kept complaining, saying that her belly with the fetus pulled her down in whichever direction she leaned with her body on the bed. She was expecting her first baby.

I immediately sent for the doctor, who fortunately happened to be at home. It didn't take him long to arrive. He also examined the mother and concluded that the fetus was dead. "What should we do now?" I asked. There was no hospital nearby, the mother's pain started to intensify, and we had no time to find a vehicle for transportation. Finding a means of transportation wouldn't have solved our problem, as transferring the patient in a carriage on these awful, unpaved roads could be fatal to her. The doctor drew me aside and said, "We have no other choice but to carry out this operation right here ourselves!" Because the fetus was already dead and the mother still had to be saved, he proposed that he would try to rotate the fetus so that its legs faced the womb and pull it out that way.

We laid the mother on a special delivery bed, disinfected our hands, and the young doctor started the operation. He was trying for a long time without any result. I asked the doctor in a whisper what was wrong. He said he didn't know, but he couldn't feel the fetus no matter where he was searching for it with his hands. I asked him to let me try to do it, knowing that I had more experience in this field than him. He quickly handed over his seat. As I intervened, I felt that the caul was still intact, though it had tightened during the contractions, which explained why we couldn't touch the fetus. Because the cervical dilation had already occurred, I broke the caul and reached the legs of the fetus. I started to pull it out slowly; and when everything seemed to be going on smoothly, I switched places with the doctor so that he could continue the operation. It went on very well for some time, but then the fetus' head got stuck. The doctor asked me again for my assistance because he couldn't manage. I pulled out the head by lifting up the fetus' trunk. Eventually, the dead body of the fetus was completely out of the womb. We both sighed in an air of relief.

Because the womb constricted reluctantly after the expulsion of the placenta, the doctor gave an injection to the patient to speed up the process. In the following week, we were nervous that the patient might develop fever, but she didn't in the end. Even nowadays, I think back with astonishment that after such a complicated operation the woman did not develop fever at all.

Part II

L ess than a week after this thrilling operation, the doctor came to my house to ask for advice concerning a new case.

"Yesterday afternoon they asked me for a delivery," he said. "I was summoned by a wealthy woman having her first delivery. She was a spoiled, only child in the family, and the parents decided that they would call a doctor instead of a midwife for the delivery. They felt that they had enough money to afford it, thinking that a delivery with a doctor would result in less pain for the expecting mother."

He explained that he was at first surprised by the idea of performing a delivery without a midwife's help, but he eventually agreed to it, nonetheless. Because it was the mother's first delivery, the process took a very long time and lasted from the afternoon until the next morning. Initially, it was only the pregnant mother who behaved impatiently during labor but later on her mother joined her too. They started to criticize the doctor for allegedly not helping the pregnant mother with the delivery, even though they were ready to compensate him for his efforts. In fact, they emphasized that they specifically did not call a midwife on the presumption that a doctor would perform the delivery in no time.

This poor doctor tried to calm them, of course, saying that the delivery was going alright. Although he said that everything was fine and the labor lasted for so long because the cervix opened too slowly, the relatives did not accept his explanation. They were expecting a miracle from a doctor.

By morning, everybody was exhausted and the baby was finally born. Because it was a big baby, a small perineal tear occurred. The doctor sewed it up; and, after being totally exhausted by all these experiences, he went home to sleep.

Sometime in the evening he went to see the patient to check up on her and see if she had developed a fever. As the doctor touched her belly, he felt that the mother's fundus of the uterus was right under her ribs, much farther up than was natural. The woman kept complaining about having severe pain. The doctor was totally clueless about the cause of the pain and hurried to my place for my help.

"Miss Mária, please tell me what is wrong here and why the womb is so enlarged. Is it possible that there is another baby left in there?" He looked at me in horror.

After I listened to the account of his observations in detail, I started to suspect the cause of the problem. "Did you ask the mother how much time has passed since she last urinated?" I enquired. He said he did not. "Then, I believe we have found the cause of her pain," I said. For during long deliveries, the urethra swells and thus the urine cannot leave the body. In this case, a catheter must be inserted because the bladder, filled with urine, pushes the womb up. "You know what! I have an idea. Since you are already here, don't go home but instead take a catheter from here that I have disinfected in boiling water. Hurry back to the patient, insert the catheter through the urethra and the mother will get better in an instant!"

The doctor came back in an hour. The broad smile on his face was noticeable from a distance. "You might not believe it Miss Mária, but as I inserted the catheter, at least two liters of urine left the body and the fundus shrank and withdrew to its place! The patient feels no pain anymore. As for me, I promised to myself that I should not be the one who sees a pregnant mother first anymore. People should instead ask for the midwife first, and if she sees any anomalies, then she can send for the doctor," the young internist said to me.

I worked for many years with this young doctor and he always asked for my advice before each case.

Later, I got word that he started to like obstetrics so much that he regularly went to practice in the town's obstetrical clinic. Since then, he became an excellent and renowned obstetrician.

WHITE LIE

Along with the many difficult hours I endured during deliveries, I also witnessed a lot of joyful cases. Among these cases there are moments that I happily recall up to this day.

Once, an old lady ran to my place, crying and shouting into the interior of my house right from the door. "Miss Mária! Come quickly, my daughter is very sick! You need to help her! We don't know the cause of the problem but she's in great pain."

"But please tell me exactly what your daughter's problem is," I said. "You know that I am a midwife, not a doctor. I am asked only to perform deliveries."

This old lady kept urging me to get prepared, saying that her daughter was expecting a baby too, in fact, but the date of delivery couldn't have arrived because her daughter had got married only seven months ago. As she recalled, she wanted to send for a doctor first to help her daughter, seeing how sick she was; but the daughter kept saying that she didn't need a doctor and she put all her trust in Miss Mária.

This excessive trust in Miss Mária seemed suspicious to me from the beginning, so I quickly got dressed, picked up my midwife's bag and followed the old lady. As we entered the premises, I heard the screaming of the young daughter from the veranda of the house. From the tone of the scream, I immediately realized that a delivery was about to take place, but I kept quiet about it to her profoundly impatient mother, who was on edge.

The young daughter was relieved when she saw me and gestured and asked me to send her mother out of the room. When we were alone, I examined her and concluded that a baby would arrive soon.

"Oh that can't be," whined the girl when I told her that she would soon become a mother. She said that despite their efforts to organize a quick wedding, it had only been seven months since she had married her husband. "What would happen if my mother and the neighbors found out that the baby came earlier than expected?" She begged me to help her and figure out something.

I went to the kitchen and asked the mother to prepare warm water to bathe a baby because her grandchild would arrive soon. I explained that her daughter was absolutely all right and it was only the beginning of the delivery for her.

"That is impossible!" The mother shouted. "The delivery can't have arrived yet; it's been only seven months since the wedding!"

"You are right, madam, the expected time of delivery has not arrived yet, but this will be a premature baby," I tried to calm her.

This, however, truly scared and unsettled her, and she said that a premature infant had to be taken to a hospital and they couldn't raise a baby like that themselves. I reassured her that there would be time to complain later, but for now she should rather heat some water for me. "We will see how everything turns out later. Nowadays, there are nicely developed premature infants that can't even be distinguished from their full-term counterparts," I tried to reassure her.

The young, expecting girl in the next room even forgot that she was in pain for quite a while as she lifted her head from the pillow and observed how I was calming down her mother.

The baby soon arrived; it was a nice, well-developed baby boy. Because there was a small perineal tear, I sent for the doctor. As soon as he arrived, the mother ambushed him in front of the door before I was able to speak to him and asked him to take the baby to a hospital immediately, because he was a premature infant.

"Premature infant?" The doctor looked at me with a query. I made a gesture and whispered in his ear that this was just partly true and wasn't the point in the case. The doctor soon realized what I meant and reassuringly touched the old lady's shoulders and said that even if her daughter's first baby came two months early, the others would certainly come properly at the ninth month.

The old lady was finally relieved. She thoroughly cuddled her grandchild. After all, a 'premature' infant really needed extraordinary care.

GYPSIES

Part I

At one time, they asked me to go to an alley of the village that was entirely inhabited by gypsies. People called it the "gypsy alley." Here, everybody knew me well since the "stork" frequented this area very often. The family which I was asked for still lived in a run-down, adobe house built into the ground. When I entered the place, I noticed with surprise that the expecting mother was lying on straw scattered on the floor. I told her husband, who stayed at the entrance, to fetch some kind of bed because it was impossible to perform the delivery in such conditions.

"Oh, I kiss your hands, nobody has a bed around here; everybody lies on the ground," he said.

"Nevertheless, the chances of infection are high," I told him. "Try to fetch a carriage so that we can take your wife to the hospital in the city."

But the woman was protesting vigorously, saying that it was out of the question that she should be taken to the hospital. She said that all the babies had been delivered on the ground without any problem; this one would be delivered too, safe and sound. Nonetheless, she asked me not to leave her side because she felt that the baby's delivery was about to take place soon. The time between contractions was getting so short that there was no time to take the mother to a hospital, and I hardly managed to at least disinfect my hands before the delivery.

I asked the husband to bring some warm water in a clean basin. This was not a simple task in the gypsy alley, and it took him quite some time to find both a basin and some water. I always had soap, a towel, and hand disinfectant in my midwife's bag and thus I used these. Then, I asked the man to fetch a blanket that I could put over the straw and under the mother. Looking at him, I realized that bringing me one was completely out of the question. He was able to bring some water but not a blanket. I didn't have a blanket either, so I decided to place my towel under the woman and laid the woman on top of it.

A nice, dark-skinned, chubby baby boy was soon born. I urged the spectators who gathered around us in the meantime to bring some clothes to the baby that we could put on him, but nobody moved. I asked the woman how they planned on dressing the baby, which she couldn't answer. Then, her husband readily offered to take off his shirt for this purpose. When he took it off, I didn't have the courage to use it, because the shirt had as many holes as Swiss cheese. Moreover, I wasn't sure about the last time it was washed as it was so dirty. I was afraid to wrap the newborn baby in it. Instead, I took off my waistcoat and used that to cover the baby.

I went to see them every day for the next week. Each time I was worried about the baby or the mother getting an infection, but eventually they turned out to be just fine.

Part II

It was with gypsies, too, that I administered the delivery of the baby of a thirteen-year-old girl for the first and last time in my life.

The gypsies certainly lead a different way of life that is based on different norms compared to ours, but whoever breaches their norms regrets it greatly.

In one afternoon, two young gypsy ladies knocked on my door and, while constantly interrupting each other, asked me to come to the 'new-building district' because the daughter of their neighbor was not feeling well. These people did not live in the gypsy alley. I asked what was wrong with the girl and why they didn't go to see a doctor if the girl was ill. "Why do you ask for me when you know that I am a midwife whose job is exclusively to perform deliveries?" I asked them.

They said they didn't know the girl's problem, but she was rolling and wailing on the floor. Her mother tried to calm her without success. They said that originally they were about to go to the doctor, but the girl started to shout that she would not let a doctor come to her side, only Miss Mária. This girl had heard about me well beforehand.

When they described the symptoms of the girl, I asked how old she was. They said she was thirteen. I had never had a case like this before; but after having been briefed about the symptoms, I was certain that the pain suggested that a delivery was about to take place. While the two ladies kept on with their explanation, I got dressed and then left with them.

As we reached the new gypsy district at the edge of the village, I noticed from a distance that a large crowd had gathered in front of the house that we were heading to.

I opened the door and saw the presumably-expecting girl lying on the floor despite the fact that there was a bed in the room. She was wailing, tearing her hair out while swearing and sending out anyone who asked her what was wrong. As I looked at her, I immediately noticed that she was pregnant. I didn't say anything to her mother, who looked at me with a query. I asked everyone including the mother to leave me alone with the girl and not to disturb us so that I could peacefully examine her. It took me some effort, especially with the mother, until I finally managed to make everyone leave the room.

When we were at last left alone, I told the girl to stop wailing so desperately since I came here to help her. I said that even though she managed to hide her secret from her parents, it would be better if she told me everything honestly. I explained that I knew she was pregnant and would soon give birth to a nice baby. My comforting voice calmed her down a bit. She looked at me and even forgot her pain for a second. Then, she said: "How did you know that I was expecting a baby when I never told it to a single person?"

To be honest, I didn't know what to reply to that for a second. Then, as I gathered my thoughts, I explained that I was Miss Mária, the local midwife as she must have known, and I helped everybody here expecting a baby. At the moment, it was she who was expecting a baby and thus I would help her now. Suddenly, she started crying again and confessed that her brother-in-law never gave her peace and kept chasing her. One time, as she recalled to me, her parents were not at home and her brother-in-law locked the doors and didn't let her leave. She was protesting and shouting, but there was nobody near to help and rescue her. After this incident, she occasionally felt dizzy, vomited a lot and when her mother asked what was wrong, she said she had an upset stomach. Her mother once noted that "it is no coincidence that this girl gained so much weight lately; she eats all the time." Nevertheless, she did not dare to inform anyone, fearing punishment. On one occasion, she felt that something had just moved inside her body. She got frightened and started to avoid everyone from this point on. Most of the time she just sat alone behind their house where nobody saw her. She wore a coat all the time so that nobody could see how much weight she had put on. She was constantly afraid that her coat might get unbuttoned and people would find out that something was moving in her belly.

"But you must have known that it couldn't stay like this forever," I said. "That baby had to be born sooner or later."

She said she didn't even think about it. She was afraid of her mother who would have beaten her to death had she found out her secret.

I decided to speak with her mother since specific things for the baby had to be prepared. I went outside and at the front of the house spotted the mother in the large crowd that had gathered around the place. I drew her aside, explained the situation and told her to prepare for the arrival of her grandchild.

Hardly had I finished the explanation when all hell broke loose. She tried to push me away to get inside and interrogate her daughter, but I held on to the door firmly. She started swearing and verbally attacking me, saying I didn't know my job and there was no one her daughter could have had a child from. I didn't mention who the father was on purpose, since otherwise people would have literally gone for one another's throats during the delivery.

I ordered her to stop swearing because the most important thing at the moment wasn't the identity of the father but to provide assistance to her daughter. When she finally realized that her daughter was really going to have a baby, she put all her curses on her daughter and on the unknown father. I said that only in case she kept quiet would she be allowed to go in the room, but if she acted recklessly she would be taken to prison. I asked her to bring warm water, to try to get some baby clothes from the neighbors, and to only come into the room if she promised not to interrogate her daughter, who had enough problems at the moment as her contractions were appearing within gradually smaller intervals.

At last, the mother left to find some baby clothes and I went inside to see the patient, who withdrew to a corner, observing the results of my previous announcement. Now that I finally managed to calm down the mother, I started the preparations for the labor. Scarcely had any time passed when the door was suddenly flung open and the mother rushed in along with her excessive verbal swearing. She said she didn't have any baby clothes ready and didn't need this bastard at all. She would kill the baby anyway after delivery no matter what. She raised the expecting girl from the bed, demanding her to disclose the identity of the father.

I called the neighbors to send somebody in who would take this miserable woman out, because she was really in the way. I knew that the time of delivery had arrived and we needed peace. Let there be peace at least until this poor girl gives birth to a baby, and then I would make sure that she along with her baby would immediately be taken to a shelter. As soon as they were in safety, the mother could discuss the ethical part of the story with her daughter's brother-in-law, later on. I hoped she wouldn't find out anything until I took the girl to a shelter.

After much suffering, a nice baby girl, weighing 2.3 kilograms (5 pounds) was born. The young mother was happy to see her pain cease and didn't seem to care about anything else from this point on. Then, thinking that she would be moved by her adorable grandchild, I let her erratic mother enter the room accompanied by two neighbors.

She calmed down a bit, but she still immediately started to interrogate her daughter to disclose the name of the newborn's father at once. The girl turned on the bed facing the wall, closed her mouth and refused to answer.

I sent them out of the room again and explained to the mother outside that her daughter needed complete peace for the next couple of days, otherwise she would develop fever. I asked her to promise me that she would not interrogate her daughter for the next three days. After that point, she could track down the father.

I was curious the next day to see whether some tragedy had happened, but everything turned out to be alright. The girl later told me that her mother kept interrogating her for some time, but seeing that she didn't answer, the mom left the girl in peace and kept her constant swearing to herself.

I managed to arrange that the girl be put right at the top of the waitlist, and she was admitted to a shelter the next day. I never found out what punishment was meted out to the brother-in-law —that is to say, to the father.

DEFYING SUPERSTITIONS

Part I

It always gave me an air of relief when I was called to a delivery and members of the family were at home, knowing that they could be sent for a doctor. On the other hand, I never liked it when the women of the neighborhood found out that childbirth was about to happen and they gathered around the place. Everybody had a better idea on how to perform deliveries.

One person advised me to lay the mother on her belly, because she herself did it that way and gave birth to a child right away. Somebody else instructed me to put the mother in hot water since in that case the delivery would happen in an instant. And there were others who suggested I remove the curse from the mother first, because with it on her, she would not be able to give birth to a child.

Every time it was so hard to convince them that the child hadn't been born yet because the time of delivery simply had not arrived. Not all babies are born in one to two hours following the first contractions; it depends on various factors.

These women, sharing suggestions, only agitated and disturbed both the mother and me. Losing one's temper during labor could become very harmful in turn. On these occasions, I entertained the thought how much easier it would be to deliver a baby in a hospital or obstetrical clinic where all these harmful kinds of advice could be avoided.

And we, local midwives, had to fight a lot against superstitions as well, especially when young couples lived together with their grandmothers! Grandparents always saw superstition everywhere. Whenever someone became ill, they would rather call a healer than a doctor.

Once, I had been checking on a family for seven days after delivery. Near the end of that week, I told the family that since both the mother and her baby looked all right and since she could now bathe her baby on her own, I would come one more day and then they would be all set. Then, the grandmother drew me aside and said that something was wrong; someone had given the baby the evil eye.[4] A woman previously came to visit them who was infamous for being capable of giving the evil eye to people. The baby had been crying all night and didn't sleep for a moment. I told her not to say such things. "If the baby cries, he simply needs something," I said. "Well, such things do exist!" the grandmother replied. She quickly got offended and said that she certainly remembered that both of her children were given the evil eye when they were young, and one of them died because of it. They called a healer to the other one. "She performed something for the baby and the curse was removed in an instant. Even though this specific healer was not as educated in midwifery as you Miss Mária, she undertook deliveries, was called to patients and could help everyone. She had a remedy for every illness," the grandmother explained.

"Do not worry, madam, we will take a look at the newborn and if some problem appears, we will bring the baby to a doctor who will help us," I told the grandmother. The old lady vigorously protested, saying that she would not let the baby be taken to a doctor. She said that if I couldn't cure the baby, she would know how to handle the situation: Three pieces of embers should be dropped in a cup of water while murmuring magic spells; the baby should drink from the cup and the remaining water should be poured out beside the baby's head. In the meantime, according to the lady, one should murmur spells and call out the name of the person who had given the evil eye to the baby. She believed that if we got the name right, the curse would go away. The only problem was that she had forgotten the spell, but she claimed that I should certainly know it.

I was frightened that they would actually make the newborn drink some liquid like that, so I removed the swaddling clothes from the baby to discover the nature of the problem. I saw that the baby had strong diarrhea. I asked the mother if she breastfed according to schedule or maybe gave the baby some extra nourishment?

She answered, with surprise, that she felt she had too much milk and thus breastfed the baby all night.

I got very angry because whenever I went to see these mothers, I told them to breastfeed their babies strictly every three hours and not at all during the night. Now we had an overfed baby. The grandmother approached us and announced that what I had just said was not correct, because feeding should not be done by an hourly schedule. The newborns knew when they were hungry and needed feeding, and they cried accordingly. I replied that maybe the grandmother, and not such a frail and tiny baby, should try eating all day and see what happened to her stomach. "There was no curse here, only a very serious upset stomach. This poor baby was crying all night because he had stomach cramps. The baby should drink only bitter tea for a while and the mother's milk should be drained. The baby could be breastfed only twice this day and every three hours tomorrow, nights excluded. If this did not help, then we must take him to the doctor," I told the people present.

The grandmother was offended and left the room with a comment that we would eventually see that she had been right about this matter. She was adamant that this baby would never get better until the curse was removed. At least, I made the young mother promise to stick strictly to my instructions.

They gave tea to the newborn but not food. The next day the mother smilingly received me saying that the baby slept nicely all night. The grandmother didn't say a word, but I saw that she only reluctantly accepted her defeat. I managed to win this time, and the young mother kept my advice, but, who knows, hadn't I visited them regularly maybe the grandmother's influence would have prevailed.

Part II

On another occasion, when I was bathing a newborn at a patient's home, a neighbor came to see me. She asked me to go to their place because their cow had been cursed by a witch. Since then, the cow only gave milk with blood in it. This neighbor's grandmother told her that for such cases a midwife was needed, for she was the only one who could help. The woman who performed the delivery of her grandmother was some sort of healer who always removed curses from them in exchange for one or two bushels of grain.

I told the neighbor woman that although I was neither a healer nor a veterinarian, I still knew that witches did not exist and there was no curse on that cow, even if it undoubtedly had some problem. "If there was blood in its milk, call a cow-specialist immediately," I said. The woman did not give in, saying there was no veterinarian in the nearby villages and asked me to at least see it myself that there was actual blood in the milk. The mother on the bed gestured that I should take a look, otherwise we would never get rid of this woman. I went to her place and because there was no milk at hand to show, she took me to the barn to milk the cow. I saw that while she was milking the first teat, the animal stayed patient, but when she moved on to a teat on the other side of the udder, the cow started kicking and milk along with blood came out.

The lady looked at me triumphantly, believing to have proved the curse. I asked her to bring a lamp because it was so dark that I couldn't see a thing in the barn. When I illuminated the udder, I noticed that there was an open wound on it that probably got torn and spilled blood during milking. I showed it to the woman to inspect how blood got in the milk. For a short moment, she looked at me with a frightened expression, but then her face got brighter and she exclaimed that "the wound was created by the curse too!"

"There is no curse here," I said. "But show me your fingers and see how long and dirty your nails are. When you milk the cow, these long nails cut the udder and the dirt infects the wound. This case is not about witchery but the lack of hygiene."

I gave her some talcum powder to put on the wound for the night. "Before milking, wash the cow's udder with warm water and rub it with butter so that the wound will not be torn forward. Your hands should always be washed before milking and your nails should be cut. If you do as I say, you'll see the cow will get better in no time and there will be no blood in the milk."

In a week, this woman came to tell me that I was right; there really wasn't any curse on that cow. She did everything according to what I said and the wound healed nicely. The cow now bore milking patiently and the milk was nice, clean and white.

Hence, a local midwife could even be a veterinarian sometimes.

CATTLE COME FIRST

Part I

After deliveries, the greatest challenge for the mothers was to patiently rest in bed during the following days. All the cattle, children, family and household chores surrounded them, and as soon as mothers delivered, they wanted to start attending to these chores. In most of the cases, deliveries took place without any complications and problems only arose later, stemming from personal irresponsibility. I always warned the mothers not to do the household chores right after delivery because they might develop a disease that could accompany them for the rest of their lives. "Leave the chores to others for some time," I would say. They always listened to me patiently, promising not to get up to do work; but nevertheless, as soon as I went away, they left their beds.

Once, I nicely and smoothly delivered a chubby baby boy. The husband did not happen to be home when the contractions started because he had gone to work in another part of the village earlier that day and was expected to return only by late night. The mother's neighbor hurried to me, saying that a delivery was about to take place. This happened around nine in the morning.

The delivery was without any complications. I bathed the baby afterwards, took care of the mother and put the newborn in a cradle next to the mother so that she could keep an eye on the newborn and also reach out to the baby from bed. I asked the neighbor to check regularly on the mother, for I had to go see another patient. I emphasized to the mother not to get up from bed because that might cause bleeding, in which case she would be helpless on her own. The neighbor promised me to take care of all the chores, even to feed the mother's pigs at noon. I told them that I would come back sometime during the evening as soon as I finished with my other patients.

First, the mother lay in bed until noon, but then she heard the pigs calling. She thought that the neighbor must have forgotten to feed them; and since she had already rested enough, she got up slowly and went to the garden. She picked a great amount of spinach that had to be pulled out from the ground with force, and so the mother's body was twitching and trembling under the pressure. Meanwhile, she started bleeding more and more but notwithstanding this decided to bring the vegetables she had collected to the pigs. She thought that once she was done feeding the animals, she would go back to bed and, hopefully, the bleeding would stop. When she reached the pig barn, she was covered in blood. Nevertheless, she started throwing the spinach to the pigs. The continuous bleeding weakened her so much that she was hardly able to reach the kitchen door where she eventually fainted.

The neighbor found her at the doorway on the ground when she came to check on her. Alone, she could hardly carry the patient back to bed, which weakened the mother's body even more. She put her in bed and hurried to me. I had just finished with one of my patients and was on my way back, when I bumped into her along the road and heard what had happened. We ran back to the house together. The mother became unconscious several times from the loss of blood. She felt dizzy and was lying as pale as a ghost on the bed. I immediately sent for a doctor. While I was waiting for him, I took the pillows from under the patient's head and put them under her legs so as to heighten them and make the womb constrict. I couldn't wait to see the doctor, who lived far from the place. He didn't have a bicycle and therefore had to come on foot, which took him a great deal of time. As soon as he got there, he examined the patient, made a salt solution and gave an injection. When the patient finally regained consciousness, her first words upon seeing us were to save her life this one time and she would never do such a thing again.

Fortunately, we managed to save the mother, but she paid a high price for her foolishness. She had to spend long months in bed, and it took a lot of time until she finally recovered.

Part II

Notwithstanding any incident, cattle always came first!

At some other night, I was called to another delivery. A man came to see me and told me to get prepared for a delivery on a farm. Her wife's contractions had already started. "Hurry up because it's my wife's second baby and this time the delivery will take less time!"

While I got dressed I asked him what farm we were going to and why we didn't use a carriage if he came so late? "This way, we will get there faster! It is not far; it shouldn't be more than two kilometers from here. We will not take the dirt roads but will rather cross straight across the fields and will get there quicker." He had both a carriage and horses, but it would have taken him much longer to take the roads with the carriage than to cross the fields. "On foot we get there faster."

From what I knew, however, that particular farm was located more than five kilometers from where I lived. As a local midwife, I was responsible for going on foot only to farms that were in a two-kilometer radius. People who called me to places farther than that were legally obliged to supply the necessary transport vehicles to reach their homes. But even though there was a regulation for that, it mostly didn't matter, because the families sometimes didn't even have food to eat, let alone a carriage or horse for transportation. And when it came to saving lives, a regulation was no excuse.

It was no use complaining about the kilometers this time either, and I departed with the man instead. It was late at night. The man brought a hand-lamp, illuminating the road in front of me, while I was following him with my essential midwife's bag. When we reached the end of the village, we went onto a field that was wet, full of bogs and had emerging muddy hills on one side and deep pits on the other. We were walking for an hour, when I realized that my clothes were completely wet and muddy because I always accidentally happened to step into the deepest puddle in the darkness. I told the man that I couldn't go any farther on this pathless field in the dark, and his lamp was of no use.

The man looked back and saw me struggling to pull one of my legs out of a pit. Seeing this, he said he would hold my hand and lead me while illuminating the ground in front of my feet. He led me from one pit to the next until we finally reached a flatter area. Here, we crossed through a sown field.

We spent another hour walking but I could notice neither a farm nor dog barking that would have signaled an inhabited area. I asked him again to tell me where they really lived, because we must have walked five kilometers by now. "We are not far," he reassured me, "but let's hurry up so that there won't be any trouble at home." We had been walking for a long time when I finally saw a tiny light in the distance.

We entered the farm. The mother was at home with only a boy around three years old. I asked the man to bring me some warm water to wash because I was covered with dirt. As I examined the mother, I noticed that the fetus was lying in a transverse position. Fortunately, I arrived at the right time. As contractions started to intensify, I helped the legs of the baby to come out and, with proper rotation, the baby was finally born, but with livid birth asphyxia. This means that the respiration was insufficient, but the heartbeats were satisfactory.

I quickly extracted saliva, gave a cold-hot bath to the baby and was soon relieved after hearing him crying. By the time I had taken care of both the mother and the baby, it was already past midnight. There was no way that I could go home at this time, and therefore they prepared a bed for me next to the patient where I lay down and slept for the night.

In the morning, I bathed the baby again and took care of the patient. I told her husband that I was supposed to come to this farm for the following eight days, but he couldn't expect me to come here on foot. It was too long a journey and I had many other patients whom I couldn't neglect. As he had a carriage with horses, I asked him to give me a ride to and from their farm.

"Then simply don't come here next time!" he told me and added that he wouldn't exhaust the horses every day on this long road. Horses had to be spared. I became angry and wouldn't have gone to them anymore hadn't I pitied the woman and her newborn. The four days following delivery are always critical as both the mother and the newborn need special attention, so I decided to walk there in the early mornings. On the fourth day, as I saw that the mother hadn't developed a fever, felt all right and had enough milk, and the baby was fine as well, I announced I wouldn't be coming back the next day and said goodbye.

The woman started to thank me, saying she knew I wasn't obliged to come this far on foot. She reassured me not to worry; she would never forget this. She said they didn't have money at the moment, but their pig was putting on fat nicely. She promised me that when the pig would have been fattened to a weight appropriate for slaughter, they would sell it and pay me for my great efforts.

This was thirty years ago, but apparently that pig is still being fattened.

MONSTROUS BIRTHS

Some less severe forms of monstrous births occurred a couple of times during my career. For example, I have encountered babies born with a cleft-lip (also called harelip), but this could be nicely corrected by plastic surgery. I also had a cleft-palate case where the baby wasn't able to suckle and thus had to be taken to a hospital. And there were some cases in which, unfortunately, even surgery couldn't offer a solution.

A young couple lived in my neighborhood who were expecting their first baby with great enthusiasm. With some excuse, they always asked me to predict how many days were left, just in case they had miscalculated something. They bought nice, elegant baby clothes and a stroller. The mother was hoping for a girl and the father for a boy, but such priorities gradually faded away as the date of childbirth approached.

Finally, the delivery was about to take place. The family members ran to my place right after the pregnant woman's first pain appeared, and the whole family gathered around their house in excitement. The woman put up with the pain surprisingly well, in spite of the fact that mothers during their first delivery are often tense and aggravated. As contractions intensified, the delivery progressed nicely. Labor didn't last long. Even though the caul was torn on time, the mother's water somehow seemed too abundant. The baby was finally born one hour after the woman's water broke.

As it is the midwife who always sees the newborn first, I was terrified when I took the first look at the baby. Initially, I didn't even know how to control my feelings so that the mother wouldn't notice my consternation. The family members were waiting in excitement for the news in the kitchen in the meantime.

I have never seen such a monstrous baby, not even in books. The baby didn't have a forehead, only a receding upper-head and two bulging eyes somewhere in-between her ears. She had a tiny, completely open back with a 2-3 centimeter hole in it revealing the spinal cord. Suddenly, I felt dizzy. The mother urged me to say if it was a boy or a girl. She wanted to see her baby at once.

I didn't mean to scare her so I covered the baby and told the mother that I couldn't show her yet, but it was a girl. "First I have to bathe the baby and show her to the doctor and only then can you have a look. It is the order of things," I tried to come up with an excuse. "Is something wrong?" she asked suspiciously. "I don't know. I cannot look after the child right now. First, I have to take care of you," I replied trying to divert the attention from the baby.

In the meantime, the placenta also got expelled, and when I saw that the patient didn't bleed more than was normal, I went to the kitchen to let the husband know that unfortunately something was wrong. His wife was fine, but the baby was born with serious deformities. He could come and take a look at the baby but should not say a word to his wife. "We will discuss what happens next, as your wife can't be distressed at the moment."

You cannot describe the disappointment on the man's face when he looked at the newborn. He really controlled his feelings, but slowly he started shedding tears. Her wife noticed it and asked what happened.

"Please don't get upset," said the husband, "but you cannot look at her. To tell the truth, this baby has deformities." Nevertheless, the mother couldn't believe him and wanted to see the baby for herself. I tried to console them, although I felt like crying too.

I sent the grandmother for a doctor because the newborn had to be taken to a hospital and couldn't stay there in that situation. When the doctor heard what the case was about, he came right away.

The newborn had seizures during the doctor's examination. The baby was already dying, and passed away soon.

It was impossible to console the mother; she was bawling uncontrollably. The doctor gave her a tranquilizing injection and tried to console them by saying that the other babies would certainly be healthy given the age of the couple. When other people had such cases, all the following babies born after the incident were healthy, he said.

I told the grandmother to collect all the baby clothes and the stroller and take them to a relative, so that they wouldn't remind the mother of this tragedy. "Don't worry, they will come in handy later!"

The mother slowly recovered, but one could tell that she was heavy-hearted whenever one saw her on the street. When we met, she lamented how bad it felt to see nice, healthy babies around the village, knowing that she couldn't have one like them. I tried to console and calm her, saying that she would also soon have a nice, healthy baby, given how young she and her husband were.

Some time had passed when, once, as I was going home from one of my patient's, somebody shouted after me to wait up. I turned around and recognized the once heavy-hearted woman from the neighborhood. She joyfully told me that she was pregnant again, although they were terrified of the upcoming delivery knowing what had happened on the last occasion. In fact, they were happy and anxious at the same time. I told her to relax because even the doctor said that the other babies would be born healthy. I suggested that she not think too much about the previous case for the sake of the baby and always try to be happy, as a mother's mood affects the fetus' development. I advised her to go on strolls, spend time in people's company and just generally have some fun.

The young woman kept my advice. She always came to visit and tell me how she enjoyed herself, how many strolls she had taken with her husband and how they were planning their future.

And so the time of delivery arrived once again. The whole street was excited about the result. Without any problem, a vivid, high-spirited boy was born who signaled his arrival with great volume. You cannot describe the joy that was present in the house. The husband almost started a dance of joy when he saw the cute, little baby. The mother was crying—this time out of joy. How different this cry was compared to last time's!

They held a large baptism. Although we didn't have to send for a doctor during the mother's second delivery, as there were no anomalies, they still invited the doctor of the village too for the event, allowing him to witness and rejoice in this vivid baby.

The baby clothes and the stroller that had been bought for the previous birth were given away to a poor family so as not to serve as reminders of the tragedy to the couple.

As for the family, they started over with a clean slate.

MIDWIFE-RHYME AT A BAPTISM

There were those rare occasions during my career when I was asked for a delivery at wealthy farmers'. Even though I was a midwife employed by the town, which basically meant that I was responsible for the poor who were allowed to use my services for free, I could still see patients in my private practice who could afford to pay the fee for my services. But the wealthy farmers that were able to pay for my services in my district numbered few, and they were rarely expecting babies.

On one afternoon, a nice, elaborate carriage stopped by in front of my house. An elderly man got out and said that he was looking for Miss Mária. "I am at your service," I said. He asked me to get dressed quickly and come to their farm, because their daughter wasn't feeling well. Her daughter's husband was not at home, and the man and her wife were already very old and didn't know the exact problem of their daughter and whether she was wailing because of her pregnancy or because of some other cause. "To tell the truth, the date of delivery has not arrived yet, but it is hard to foresee it, because it will be the second baby of our daughter. She already has a little girl," he told me.

Finally, I could take a comfortable, nice carriage to a patient's place. This was a rather uncommon event in my profession, because the families I frequented often didn't even have food to eat let alone a carriage. Therefore, I was accustomed to walking four or five kilometers in freezing weather, snow or mud.

This farm was far away as well, but with the carriage we quickly reached it. It felt like the horses were flying on the way. We entered the farm through a poplar tree alley. There were a lot of cattle around the house and many barns too. It was surrounded by hundreds of acres of farmland, as I was later told. The old man worked on the farm with his son-in-law.

When I entered the room, I saw the mother and a young lady from the neighboring village bustling around the pregnant woman. They were relieved when they saw me. They said they had sent for me specifically because they had heard so many good things about my midwife activity. Although they knew that I was a community midwife, and that there was also another midwife with a private practice in the district, from what they had heard they had more trust in Miss Mária. "Well, trust is half-success," I thought to myself. I sent everybody out of the room so that I could examine the patient. Everything was prepared in advance: warm water, basin, soap, nice clean towels and baby-clothes.

In my experience, poor women generally bore the pain of labor better. I even had a poor, pregnant mother who gave birth to a baby without a single wail. This young mother, on the other hand, lived in a wealthy family and took childbearing with the according temperament. She was tense and disorderly. She was shouting, wailing and tossing herself all over the place. I could hardly examine her. Contractions took place every two or three minutes. The heartbeat of the fetus sounded odd to me. Sometimes the sounds came from the left, sometimes from the right side of the mother's belly, like an echoing sound in the womb. Because the patient was tossing herself on the bed impatiently and the caul was torn in the meantime, I could no longer listen to the heartbeat.

The labor went on well and soon a nice little boy was born. What a joy it was that after their girl, they now had a boy to be the heir of the family. They always wanted a boy so that somebody could cultivate the lands in the future. When I was taking care of the baby, I was also looking out for the placenta to get expelled. I was waiting, but nothing happened. Then, I noticed that the size of the mother's belly was still quite substantial. It was suspicious; I was looking for a heartbeat again, and found it. We were about to have twins here, I thought to myself, but I didn't want to let the mother know because she was lying on the bed so relieved after her pain had ceased.

I went out to see the grandmother, who had gathered a small crowd to rejoice in her grandson's birth. I whispered to her to get prepared for another grandchild. I asked her to send someone for a doctor because her daughter would soon start feeling pain again. Even if no problem occurred in the end, it was always handy to have a doctor for a twin delivery, just in case.

She got so frightened by the news that she didn't send anyone for a doctor and instead started running around the farm, complaining that her daughter could not endure another delivery. Although she forgot her task, when I hurried back to the patient I had the reassuring feeling that a doctor was supposedly being on his way. The patient had new contractions. She got scared and didn't understand why she was in pain again. I explained that this pain was natural and advised her not to get scared but be happy about her twins. She instead started wailing loudly, saying she was so weak she couldn't give birth to another child. Trying to encourage her, I said this labor would not last as long as the previous one. The caul was soon torn and a new baby was delivered, who again turned out to be a boy.
Hearing the boy's screaming, the grandmother rushed into the room to see what was going on. When she saw that another baby was born without any complications and they had two grandsons now, she suddenly realized that she had forgotten to send for a

doctor. I became very frustrated, as I was expecting a doctor to step into the room at any moment during the delivery, but she hadn't even sent for one. Her daughter's life could have been at risk because of it. Fortunately, there were no complications; the placenta got expelled properly and there was no excessive bleeding. As we finished bathing both babies it had already been past midnight. They didn't want me to leave and therefore prepared a bed for me next to the mother where I slept for the night.

The post-delivery period for staying in bed passed without any major problems or even fever for the mother. Six days after delivery the young woman was already walking outside. The babies had good appetites and the mother had plenty of milk. They were baptised two weeks after the delivery.

I had never been at such an impressive baptism before, even though I was invited to a lot of newborns' baptisms during my profession. This one in particular might have been as planned as a wedding-party. There were a hundred guests invited, and all the godparents were wealthy farmers too. An actual queue of carriages accompanied us to the event.

There was a huge lunch at noon. All the rooms were opened, connecting the whole building together into one giant place, and tables were set up inside. When the guests took their seats, the grandfather asked me to sit in the center between the two godparents. Before the food was served, the grandfather whispered in my ears, "Miss Mária, please place a platter on the table for the honorary fee and perform the 'midwife-rhyme' for the guests!" I looked at him in astonishment. I didn't even know there was such a thing as a "midwife-rhyme" let alone performing one right there. "Well, this is a tradition here," the grandfather tried to encourage me and said that it was going to be alright; he would teach me the lines. He sat next to me, started reciting the verse slowly and asked me to repeat it after him. "This must be done," he said, "because all the guests are awaiting it."

The excitement I felt could be compared to what I was feeling during the first delivery I performed in my career. I put a platter on the table, then the grandfather started to whisper the lines in my ear. The guests had fun when they saw what a bad apprentice I was. Then, to avoid further embarrassment, I started reciting the following text:

"Nagy utakat, vidéket bejártam,
Míg ezekre a kisfiúkra rátaláltam.
Elszakadt a bocskorom talpa,
Pénzért varrta meg a varga.
Mivel az én zsebem lyukas,
Nem áll meg benne a garas,
Azért ezt a tál helyettesíti."
"Great roads, lands I've wandered around,
Until finally these babies I've found.
My bootstrap was torn on the way,
A cobbler repaired it for pay.
As my pocket is full of holes,
It does not hold any coins,
Thus this platter will replace it."

When I finally finished the verse, I was more exhausted than a mother after labor. Hardly had I caught my breath when I noticed the money overflowing from the platter. I received several months' pay there. When the grandfather brought the platter to me, he had a huge smile on his face and said, "You see, it was worth reciting the midwife-rhyme after all."

After this performance, the lunch finally started. We had chicken soup, stuffed cabbage, roasted chicken, schnitzel, different side dishes, vegetables and compotes. Then, we had a cake, freshly baked pastries and delicious, quality wines.

The celebration ended late at night, after which I was taken home in a carriage. They gave me a decent amount of the leftover dishes to take home to my daughter. They were so grateful that the delivery took place smoothly and without any complications that they didn't know how to show their gratitude.

This is how once in my life I attended the delivery of wealthy people's babies.

OUR TIME IN THE AMBULANCE

In olden days, women used to deliver babies at home, as it wasn't required to give birth at a hospital or obstetrical clinic. A doctor was rarely present at these deliveries. Even if there was one residing in the village, he was seldom at home, rather paying visits to patients at their places. Therefore, midwives bore more responsibility. We had to be prudent not to send for the doctor either too late or too early, so as not to waste the doctor's time, while simultaneously trying not to endanger the life of the mother or her newborn.

How much I hesitated during each delivery whether I should send for a doctor immediately or wait just a little longer to see the situation unfold! Modern obstetricians who work at comfortable, well-equipped obstetrical clinics and hospitals and who attend deliveries in the presence of other doctors cannot even imagine what it meant for a midwife to perform a delivery in the old days. For instance, a midwife needed all her composure, ingenuity and competence to perform a delivery on her own at a farm, having only oil lamps, poor medical equipment and for the most part no medicine or doctor at her disposal.

The following case illustrates what difficulties I had to endure until a doctor arrived at last.

One day, a pregnant woman sent her neighbor to ask me to go to their farm, because her contractions had started. This was at the time when I already owned a bicycle and, weather permitting, could use it to travel faster. Nevertheless, it still often happened that I had to carry my bike on my back on my way home from a delivery because the rain made the dirt roads so muddy that my bike would get stuck on them. Fortunately, the weather was nice this time and I quickly reached the place by bike. The pregnant woman's husband wasn't at home, only her mother. I examined the patient; she was having her first delivery and had painful contractions. I immediately noticed that she had edema in her legs, and her skin was swollen around her eyes as well. I asked if she had seen a doctor regarding the disease. She said no, because the doctor lived far from this farm. She was afraid to see him anyway because her neighbor said that a potential examination would allegedly involve compressing her body which, in turn, would hurt the fetus. Her friend in the neighborhood reportedly had a smooth delivery last time, and she had never been examined by a doctor either.

"Well, the fact that you haven't seen a doctor is of great concern," I said, "because your kidneys might not be functioning properly and that's why your legs are so swollen. Consequently, this might cause complications during delivery." I quickly did a urine test that revealed high levels of protein. I was frightened that this woman might get seizures during delivery, which I couldn't deal with myself, and thus a doctor had to be sent for. But, of course, the usual question came up again: who should be sent for a doctor since the grandmother was so old she couldn't go to the next village on foot? I asked her to try to go to the next farm at least where the owners had a carriage with horses and ask them to take my message to the doctor. I gave her a letter describing the situation that should be given to the doctor.

When the grandmother left, I went to the kitchen to get a wooden cooking spoon to have something in hand in case the mother got her first seizure. In such cases, it was advised to put a wooden spoon in the mother's mouth so that she wouldn't bite her tongue.

The grandmother eventually managed to find a farm with a carriage and people to carry the letter. Unfortunately, these people didn't find the doctor at home. Although they were told which farm the doctor was supposed to be at, the people carrying my message instead waited at the doctor's house. They were afraid that they would accidentally bypass him on the way should they leave his place. Nonetheless, the doctor didn't seem to be coming. In the meantime, I was becoming more and more impatient as I was looking outside the window for them to arrive. Suddenly, I noticed that the patient's body straightened and her mouth became so forcefully stiff that I could hardly put the wooden spoon in it. She was having her first seizure.

When the seizure ended, I finally heard a carriage stopping in front of the house and was relieved when I was told that they had managed to bring the doctor. He examined the patient and told me that from my letter he suspected that the patient would need to be hospitalized and therefore he had already asked for an ambulance. Unfortunately, the only ambulance in the city was being used, and thus he left a message to come to the farm as soon as it became available.

The poor woman suffered another seizure, but, at least, now the doctor was here to help. We were anxiously waiting for the ambulance. At last, it arrived and the doctor asked me to accompany the patient inside the ambulance car. He had other urgent cases to attend to and new seizures of the pregnant mother were likely to take place on the way with which the grandmother would not be able to deal.

There were only a driver and a nurse in the ambulance, but not a doctor. They sat in the front and I was sitting in the back with the patient. The contractions started to intensify. I urged the driver to speed up, but he could only drive slowly on that bad, gravel road. He was already exhausted by the time he got to the farm, as his shift should have ended a long time ago. He told me that he was the ambulance's sole designated driver and he had been continuously on duty since last night because they had received so many calls. He was hardly able to stay awake, he kept nodding off. He was afraid he might fall asleep.

When he could no longer keep his eyes open, he told me that we would stop driving for ten minutes in order for him to rest a bit and recharge himself. I told him and the nurse that we shouldn't stop now, if possible, because every minute could make a difference for the mother. This was the moment when the nurse offered to drive the car so that the driver could get some sleep in the meantime.

I can't say I was content with this change of roles, but I kept this thought to myself knowing that at least we would keep going. Naturally, I couldn't pay much attention to what happened in the front of the car because the mother's contractions intensified and she started wailing. In the meantime, I was staying steady with the wooden spoon in my hand, anticipating another seizure. The nurse was driving smoothly for a while, but then suddenly a horse-drawn carriage entered the road from a path that was concealed by dense trees. When the nurse driving the car noticed the carriage heading our way, in order to avoid a collision, she turned the steering wheel so that it caused the car to make a huge jump and then lean in the direction of the ditch on the side of the road. The sleeping driver woke up immediately to this turn of events and by instinct, being still half-asleep, grabbed the wheel and turned it in the opposite direction. This was a mistake, for the car now leaned with all its mass the other way. Fortunately, it did not turn over, but this sudden change of direction made the patient fall off the bed and me on top of her. The poor woman stopped her wailing from the shock. I was careful to throw away the wooden spoon in advance so as not to damage the mother with it. I even paid attention not to hurt the mother's belly and the baby in it.

The driver stopped the ambulance and ran to the back to see if we were all right. My body was so entangled with that of the mother that the driver could hardly untangle us. Luckily, apart from the shock, we were just fine.

As we were getting closer to the hospital, the mother bore her pain less patiently and hardly had we reached the hospital when her labor began. A nice strong boy was born through a demanding delivery. We were all relieved that it went well because everybody was anxious that the baby might have been hurt during the accident.

Later on, the mother left the hospital and came to see me with her baby at my home and we laughed together about our time in the ambulance. She kept wondering what we might have looked like in the back of the ambulance on the floor, entangled with each other—after all, the driver had looked at us with such a weird expression on his face.

DEATH

During my 28-year practice as a midwife, I even encountered the death of a mother once. It is always a tragedy for a family when their baby dies before or after delivery; but when the mother dies, it amounts to a trauma.

This time, I attended the delivery of an experienced mother. I didn't notice any anomalies during labor, and a nice, healthy baby girl was born in a short time. Everybody was very content —especially the mother, since it was her first girl after delivering many boys. The mother's pain ceased after delivery and she started telling me anecdotes joyfully while I was bathing her baby.

After I finished bathing her, I swaddled the baby and checked the mother again to see whether she was bleeding more than usual after labor. To my surprise, there was a pool of blood under her on the bed and her body was still bleeding. I quickly put a cold compress on the mother and told her that I would send someone for a doctor who would give an injection to resolve the problem. The relatives had arrived in the meantime. All of them advised me what should be done to stop the bleeding, but they didn't even want to hear about a doctor. Even the patient rejected it, saying everything would be fine.

Nevertheless, as the patient was busy seeing her relatives, I drew her husband into the kitchen and asked him to go for the doctor. "There's no need to tell the relatives or the mother where you are going. Let's not upset them!" I told him. The husband almost started to argue saying that a doctor was not necessary and we shouldn't trouble ourselves about it. I kept insisting and didn't give in. I quickly wrote a few lines and asked him to take it to the doctor and return with him.

Fortunately, the doctor happened to be at home and came to see us right away. He thoroughly examined the patient and her placenta to see whether it had been expelled properly. He found everything all right, but the bleeding would not seem to stop. He gave an injection to the patient and stayed, instead of going home. The womb constricted, but the mother kept on bleeding. The doctor told me that he was going to disinfect his hands and examine the vagina to see if there was a uterine rupture. He found a small rupture that he constricted with clips, but the bleeding, nevertheless, did not want to cease.

The patient had already lost a lot of blood, so the doctor gave her a saline solution; however, the bleeding continued.

"We have no other choice," he said, "but to constrict her abdominal arteries." Together, we carefully lifted the patient and placed the doctor's tool under the waist and over the belly around her body. Then, we constricted the arteries and the bleeding actually stopped. The doctor and I were somewhat relieved, but the patient started to wail and scream. She was in so much pain that she begged us to loosen the constriction. As we loosened it, the bleeding started again.

We had to constrict the abdominal arteries again because the bleeding started to intensify. The patient couldn't take the pain anymore. She wailed so loudly that the relatives came in to ask us several times to relieve her. The doctor came back one more time at nine o'clock in the evening. We stayed optimistic even after midnight. He gave an injection and a salt solution to the patient again, but they were of no use. We became completely baffled by this case. The patient passed away at four o'clock in the morning;

she was a nice, 43-year old gypsy lady.

I felt really sorry for her. She was such a decent lady. I had known her for a long time, and now she had to leave her little newborn girl, to whom she had been looking forward to so much after all her boys.

We were waiting for the report of the autopsy because we couldn't figure out the cause of the bleeding. Then, we learned that the mother had visited the hospital many times before with bleeding problems. The doctors even wanted to operate on her; but, since she was in the second month of her pregnancy, they postponed the operation until the post-delivery period. This poor lady had cancer.

Because the woman's pain ceased during childbearing, she did not see a doctor and still managed to deliver her baby. During labor, however, the cancerous tumor started to bleed, which was fatal at this point. If we had had cancer screening programs at that time and they had discovered the tumor in time, they might have been able to save her life—but this way it was all too late.

I delivered many babies in this neighborhood, and I saw that the deceased mother's relatives brought up her baby girl. When she grew bigger and was playing on the street, she always addressed me when passing by, "Miss Mária, who are you visiting this time?" My heart always broke on these occasions, and I recalled how much her poor mother rejoiced in having her first girl.

THE MOTHER,
THE MIDWIFE AND
THE DRIVER

One could never forecast the actual date of a delivery, not to mention the fact that women gave birth to children wherever they happened to be. These circumstances always created an atmosphere of randomness and unpredictability.

One day, a woman came to my place to inform me that on a neighboring farm there was a newlywed wife who wanted to deliver her baby at an obstetrical clinic, but she couldn't predict the date of delivery herself. She wanted to go to the clinic neither too early nor too late. Consequently, I was asked to visit and consult with her when I had some time.

I told this woman to tell the young wife to head to town and ask for advice in the clinic itself. "She cannot do that," the woman replied. "Her husband leaves home for work during the day and she has to stay at the farm. They have a lot of cattle to attend to and the town is far away. Nevertheless, could you please see her, examine her and try to estimate the date of delivery," she asked me. "This way, she could go to the clinic on time and ask her husband to stay home with the animals."

I kept explaining to her that this was too risky. If the first contractions started, childbirth could follow in a matter of hours. Prediction of the approximate date is never reliable and can be off by one or even two weeks.

"Oh, there is more than a month remaining until the delivery!" She reassured me and asked me again to go to see the young woman on the farm because, even though she couldn't come with me to the farm, the pregnant mother was expecting me at her home and wanted to discuss other matters as well.

It was still early in the morning, the weather was nice, I had just finished checking on my other patients, so I thought I might pay a visit to this woman and explain to her that deliveries did not work the way she thought they did. I biked to her place without even bringing my midwife's bag, thinking, after all, I was only invited for a conversation.

As I was approaching the farm, I found it far too deserted. I couldn't see anyone around. Because the dog was on a chain and the kitchen door was wide open, I entered the house. I couldn't find anyone in the kitchen either. I said 'good day' loudly, to which a voice in the next room replied, asking me to come in. I was surprised to see the mother lying in bed. I asked her what the problem was. She said she didn't know, but she had felt such acute pain twice that day that she had to lie down for a while. She got scared being alone and was very relieved when she heard my voice. She was digging up plants in the garden, which must have caused her pain.

I disinfected my hands, examined her and concluded that contractions had started. I wasn't sure what to do. I hadn't brought my midwife's bag, since, initially, I was invited only to give advice, thinking that there was more than a month remaining until delivery.

I said I would go home on my bike to fetch my midwife's bag

and then come back as soon as I could, because the delivery had started. "Oh, please don't leave me here on the farm alone!" she begged me. She said she didn't want to deliver at home but at an obstetrical clinic. She would write a few sentences to her husband, leave the message on the table, get dressed quickly and I could take her to the clinic. She said the contractions were not intense and we could still make it on time. On the main road there were usually so many carriages passing that we could just ask a driver to take us to the clinic in exchange for some money.

In those days, hardly any women wanted to have a delivery in a clinic; they would rather stay home. Finally, I had a young woman who wanted to go to a clinic at all costs and I wasn't sure if we could make it.

I was not content with her idea, but I understood that it was still a better solution to accompany the patient than to leave her completely alone on the farm. Since it was her first pregnancy, I thought we might even make it to the clinic on time provided we could catch a ride.

The young woman got dressed quickly and we left. The clinic was located about five kilometers from the farm. Even for a healthy person, this journey would have taken at least an hour on foot. I hoped to see a car passing by that could give us a lift. I still considered it possible that the delivery could drag on for an hour and we could make it to the clinic.

She didn't speak on the way; I was pushing my bike and she was walking beside me. Sometimes, when she had to slow down or pause, she ground her teeth and could hardly keep herself from wailing. She clearly wanted to make it to the clinic, so she tried to hold her act together.

Then, I heard a horse-drawn carriage approaching us from behind. I told the young woman not to say anything, just leave the talking to me. I didn't mean to tell the driver that the mother was just about to have her delivery in case he got afraid and wouldn't let the mother get in. I advised her to pull her coat together and step aside.

A man, around 22 years of age, drove the empty carriage. I stopped him and explained that this young woman didn't feel well and asked him if he could give her a ride. He picked her up without a comment, and I started following them on my bike.

The carriage unsurprisingly jolted up and down the road full of potholes. I was riding my bike slowly, directly behind the carriage and was keeping an eye on the woman. I saw that she started grinding her teeth more often. She managed to bear her pain quietly up to a point, but then all of a sudden she couldn't hold it in anymore and let out a high scream.

The driver looked back in shock to see what happened. The mother then screamed out even higher. The man quickly stopped the carriage, got off and walked to the back to ask what was going on here. I admitted that this young lady would soon deliver a baby and we were heading to the obstetrical clinic. I asked him kindly to help us and take us to the clinic quickly because every minute counted.

Hearing this he started swearing in an elaborate Hungarian way, claiming that we had fooled him a great deal. He had never seen a delivery, and had he known the real nature of the situation he wouldn't have taken us in his carriage. I knew this very well, but I also understood that necessity knew no law. I told him that it was no place for a debate now and we should rather carry on. I asked him to drive fast but slow down whenever he heard the woman wailing. The man kept on swearing but nevertheless got back onto the carriage and whipped the horses. In revenge, he warned us not to count on him during delivery; he said he would rather leave us alone without a horse or carriage than help us. I reassured him that he wouldn't have to do anything except drive those horses faster.

The wailing of the mother started to intensify and I asked the man to stop and let me get into the carriage. I took my bike up with me and stayed at the mother's side. Hardly had we gone four kilometers more than I saw that the mother's labor pains had begun. Oh my god, how greatly I wished she held out just for one more kilometer and not to have the delivery in the carriage! I asked the driver again to slow down a bit, but he kept swearing loudly and whipped the horses even more. I ordered him vehemently to stop his continuous swearing, because the poor woman and I had ample problems at the moment and he was only disturbing us. Hearing this, he finally slowed down a little. When I saw that the woman had managed to relax a bit between two contractions, I allowed the driver to speed up again. The man stayed silent for some time, but then he started his speech over, demanding that the woman avoid delivering in the back.

As the wailing and swearing intensified, we finally reached the clinic. A nurse was standing outside. I asked her to come quickly and help us to lift the mother off the carriage and take her into the clinic.

The driver hastily jumped off the carriage, took out my bicycle and leaned it to the wall of the building. No sooner had we lifted the mother out of the carriage than he jumped back on it and whipped the horses. He didn't even say good luck, just rode away. "Well, this man won't give a woman a ride again either," I thought to myself.

We reached the obstetrical ward with the parturient woman. There, the lady on duty could help us. We laid the patient on a bed and were about to undress her, but it turned out that there was no time for that. She gave a sharp scream and her baby was soon born. She was a nice, big baby girl.

The mother and her baby were both healthy and left the clinic after eight days. They were very happy with each other.

Afterwards, we laughed a lot with the mother about the story of her baby's birth and kept saying that she was uniquely delivered by three people: the mother, the midwife and the driver.

EVEN DOCTORS LISTENED TO ME

Part I

An obstetrical clinic was opened in the neighboring village. Although it consisted of only two rooms, one for deliveries and the other for mothers—in the latter there were only three beds altogether for patients—it was still a special clinic designated for expecting mothers.

The clinic didn't have a permanent staff and thus the local doctors and midwives held shifts regularly. They even installed a telephone inside the building. The delivery room was well-equipped, and unlike at homes, childbirths took place in sterile conditions there. That is to say, they could have taken place, for even our three-bed capacity was usually empty. Although this clinic meant a great deal to us, and we did everything to attract women, our efforts remained all in vain. It is interesting to note that even in the beginning of the 1940s women were afraid of "clinical deliveries." Everybody wanted to deliver at home. This was an ancient, instinctual distrust. They thought that delivery at a clinic meant death, and delivery at home meant survival.

I was on duty at this clinic one day when a young woman already feeling her labor pains was brought in. I disinfected my hands and prepared everything for the delivery. Contractions had started by this time, and soon a nice, healthy girl was born. When the placenta got expelled, I noticed a small perineal tear. I called the doctor on the phone to come in—what a handy tool it was! He wasn't at home, so I left him a message. He arrived thirty minutes later; and, since it was only a small tear, he sutured it with three stitches and thus solved the problem quickly. He examined the mother and the baby and found no anomalies, so he went home.

Apparently, even our local doctor cared about the good reputation of the clinic. Despite the fact that complications requiring a doctor's presence did not always occur, he still came in to see the patients every day.

The mother with the perineal tear developed a fever the next day. In those times, medicines were not as effective as they are today, but the doctor still gave her an injection. By the third day she had developed a high fever and we couldn't figure out its cause. Once again, we tried to think about what might have gone wrong in this seemingly perfect delivery. The caul was torn properly thirty minutes before delivery and we didn't have to intervene. We had sewn the perineal tear in sterile conditions. The doctor disinfected both his hands and the area of the wound. Hence, we acted in the most careful manner, but then what could have gone wrong?

The doctor examined the wound once again, but it wasn't even red or swollen so there could be no inflammation. Even though the patient received only food that was easy to digest and we also tried giving her a purgative, her body temperature was thirty-nine degrees Celsius and it didn't look like it was about to go down.

By the fourth day, she was regularly shivering, followed by a feeling of hotness of such intensity that she threw off all blankets of various sizes. Her temperature reached forty-one degrees by the night and she started to shiver again, making the bed shake along with her. We put warm clothes on her and yet she kept shivering. When it stopped, the heat came back. In the latter case, we washed her body with wet clothes and put cold compresses near her heart. Nothing seemed to help.

This case puzzled us so deeply that the doctor didn't go home but stayed at the clinic and kept walking up and down the corridor. "What are we supposed to do, Miss Mária?" he asked. "We are helpless and this patient is going to die!"

I kept on thinking about the potential cause of the problem; and then, out of the blue, an idea popped into my mind. I told the doctor that as the saying goes 'two heads are better than one,' so he might just call in another doctor from the city hospital. He looked at me, didn't say a word, went to the phone, called the obstetrical clinic of the city hospital and asked an obstetrician to come to our place at once by car; he would take care of the costs.

An obstetrician arrived from the city in two hours. He also thoroughly examined the patient and asked both her and us about the sequence of events during delivery. He couldn't find any cause either that could explain this high fever.

He was still thinking about the cause when he asked the patient to open her mouth. She opened it wide from her astonishment. The doctor looked inside and asked, "How long have you had so many bad teeth?" "Well," the patient replied, "some time now; but I didn't see a dentist because my neighbor suggested that I not have them fixed during pregnancy, especially not have them pulled out, because that would harm the baby."

"Well, I believe we have found the cause then!" the doctor exclaimed. "These teeth should have been taken care of. Pus filled the roots of the bad teeth, and this pus entered the bloodstream after delivery, which in turn caused the high fever."

He quickly called for an ambulance that took the patient to the hospital. They kept her there for a long time, treated her teeth and thus managed to save her life.

Part II

Local midwives were occasionally asked to be on duty at the gynecology clinic of the city hospital if necessity dictated and they were low on staff. Once, I was asked to do a night shift. They specifically brought my attention to a patient who had an operation for a cancerous tumor. They didn't know what to do with her because she was vomiting repeatedly. They gave her only liquids, like milk, tea, and soup, but she always vomited them up. This poor patient became so weak that her life began to be on the line.

The head doctor tried everything, but they couldn't manage to keep a single drop of any given liquid in the patient's body; and, seeing this constant vomiting, they also started to worry for the patient's life. They tried giving her several medicines, but she kept vomiting them up. Although she was thirsty as a camel and could have drunk liters of liquid, her body didn't want to store a drop of it. She vomited up the exact same amount she had drunk.

I entered the ward and observed the patient. She really was in a dreadful condition. As soon as she noticed the new nurse on duty, she asked for a drink. Scarcely had I given her some tea than she started to vomit.

In the meantime, the head physician also asked me to come by his office where he told me to pay special attention to this patient. He asked me to constantly keep an eye on the patient and phone him at home in case anything happened. The doctor and I had known each other for a long time, but I had never seen him so worried until that point. He seemed to be very disturbed by the condition of the patient. "Even though the patient went through a successful operation, we can't help her now because of her constant vomiting. Sadly, this poor woman is possibly going to die," he sighed.

Suddenly, an idea came to my mind. I hesitated for a moment about whether to speak up in the doctor's presence, because he had a reputation of being a rather strict and quick-tempered man and all the other midwives were afraid of him. Everybody knew him as an excellent expert in his field, but he didn't tolerate any disagreement concerning his issued directives. But after all, the life of a patient was on the line, so I decided to share my thoughts.

"This patient must have an extraordinarily nervous stomach. She feels extremely thirsty and her stomach is empty; but the way I heard it, the clinic allows her to drink up to even half a liter of liquid at a single time. This is not right! Her nervous stomach twitches after it receives such a high volume of liquid and rejects it right away. I suggest we give the patient a tablespoon of ice-cold milk every hour. This small amount of cold milk will cool and calm the stomach and won't induce ejection. Not to mention that the milk will also nourish her," I told the doctor.

The head doctor listened to me and without a reply grabbed my hand and pulled me into the ward. We stopped at the patient's bed and the doctor announced that I would be on duty this night and give her exactly one spoonful of ice-cold milk every hour but not more than that, strictly one spoonful per hour. The doctor warned other people too not to give this patient any liquid, no matter how much she begged for it, because her life depended on it. He had to go home then.

I had many things to attend to that night but still managed to show up every hour at the side of the patient's bed, armed with one tablespoon of milk. This poor woman was shaking from thirst when she noticed me with the milk. She always begged me to give at least one more spoon of milk, but I stuck to the amount despite my pity for her. She once grabbed my hand, seized the spoon and started to lick it hoping to find some remaining drops of milk on it.

When her body didn't eject the first spoon of milk, my hopes started to rise. She didn't vomit the next spoon of milk either. By then, she started to have high hopes too and stayed up all night, keeping an eye on the clock and calling me desperately as soon as I was a second late.

The head doctor apparently didn't seem to be able to fall asleep that night either, because he phoned me at one o'clock in the morning, asking how my plan was working out. When I told him that the mother's life was probably saved because she didn't vomit a single time, the doctor kept quiet for some time. There was a long silence at the other end of the line and then he softly uttered, "All right Miss Mária, thank you!" and hung up the phone.

The doctor arrived at the hospital early in the morning of the following day. He first visited me and when he heard that I was still giving the one tablespoon of milk every hour to the patient and she didn't vomit it up, he entered the ward quite serenely. He instructed us to keep up this amount.

The patient started to get back her spirit during the following days and also started to take some food. Because her operation had been successful, she slowly regained her strength and was released from hospital in ten days' time.

Later on she often remarked that a tablespoon of ice-cold milk had brought her back to life.

DAY OF THE TWINS

It was always a great experience for both the mothers and me to attend the deliveries of twins. Notwithstanding the increased risk of complications in these deliveries, I was happy to perform them.

One day, I was assigned to be on duty at the obstetrical clinic I mentioned before. When I began my shift, a mother and her newborn twins were already at the clinic. I was watching her two beautiful boys when I was told that they had just brought in a new pregnant mother. I was glad to hear it, knowing that after not using our full capacity for so long, two out of the three beds at the clinic would finally be occupied. The mothers had a lot of services available to them at the clinic, yet, as mentioned before, they were reluctant to have their deliveries here.

I examined the newly admitted woman and noticed heartbeats coming from both sides of her belly. I asked her where she felt the baby moving. She replied both upwards and sideways. "It is quite a rare occasion, but we will have twins here!" I said.

I phoned the doctor and asked him to come in and examine the patient in case any complications might arise later during the night when we wouldn't be able to reach him. He examined the patient right after he arrived and concluded that we were expecting twins indeed.

The caul was soon torn and a boy was born an hour later. The doctor examined him and said that this baby was so small that we should expect another one. The mother's belly stayed increased in size and we could still clearly listen to a baby's heartbeat in the womb. The mother started to accept the idea that another baby was soon to come. New contractions started in about ten minutes and the caul was torn again. This baby, compared to the previous one, was born with his legs coming out first, and thus the doctor's presence proved to be essential in the end. This baby turned out to be a boy too. The placenta got expelled nicely and everything seemed to be fine. The doctor stayed there for some time; when he saw that everything was all right, he went home.

At eleven o'clock that night they reported bringing in another pregnant woman at the clinic and asked me to hurry because the mother's contractions were very intense. I didn't have time to examine the patient and could hardly disinfect my hands because contractions were going on and the caul was torn. A baby girl was soon born. I told the mother what a beautiful girl she had. She replied that she would have preferred a boy since she already had a girl, but obviously she was very content with another girl too. She was particularly happy with being through with the delivery.

This newly born baby weighed only two kilograms, even though the size of the mother's belly suggested a larger baby upon arrival. This case became suspicious. I examined the mother again and was stunned: I was listening to a distinct heartbeat of another baby from the belly. "These must be twins as well," I thought to myself.

I ran to the telephone and called the doctor. "Come quickly, someone is having twins again!" It was late at night and obviously I had woken him up. He asked me, being still half-asleep, not to play jokes on him. "Not all pregnant women will deliver twins today. You must be so into delivering twins that you start to see them everywhere," he said. "But doctor, I clearly hear another baby's heartbeat," I said, "so please do come in!"

He soon arrived at the clinic. By that time the mother's contractions had started again. Her second baby in the womb was lying in the so-called transverse position. The doctor quickly disinfected his hands so that he would be ready by the time the caul was torn. He easily managed to change the position of the baby, who was soon born. To the greatest joy of the mother, he turned out to be a boy. It was the mother's first boy.

The doctor stayed with us for a while, and when he saw that everything was alright, he went back home. Leaving the place, he jokingly said, "There were three twin deliveries today, so we are out of free beds. Please, Miss Mária, do not schedule any more twins for today!"

Needless to say, everybody was fascinated by the twins; they were so adorable, all in one place. They were developing nicely, except for one of the boys who had to be fed with hand, because he was so weak he wasn't able to suckle. We continually put warm water bottles around him. In ten days, they grew sufficiently strong so we could let them leave the clinic. Later, I was anxious to see all of them survive.

Once, I was walking down the street and saw a woman coming in front of me leading twins. I was inspecting how cute the children were, when I heard that their mother whispered in their ears to say 'good day' to Miss Mária. This was the point at which I recognized the woman. She was the one who had delivered the two frail babies at our 'day of the twins' at the clinic. Her children had become quite healthy and lovely by now. We met several times afterwards and the twins no longer needed help in this respect; they instantly recognized me and said 'good day' on their own.

PASSIONATE LOVE OF A HUSBAND

It is often said that spouses are initially bound together by love and later by their children. In my opinion, spouses rather are truly bound together by empathy and mutual respect.

Once, I was on duty at the clinic when a young couple arrived. The contractions of the young woman had visibly started, and thus I asked her husband to say goodbye to his wife. "You can go home and your wife and I will go into the delivery room. Tomorrow, you can come to see the baby," I told him.

"You can't be serious about leaving my wife at this crucial moment! Not in a million years!" he replied. He announced strong-mindedly that he wouldn't allow his wife to be taken away without him at her side. He loved his wife a great deal and had promised not to leave her alone regardless of any situation. On top of these reasons, the husband complained that he surely would not survive this delivery. "Calm down," I reassured him, "you are the one who will most certainly survive, but please let us do our job! I must examine your wife right now. If you truly love her as you say, you will leave her with me for the time of the delivery and won't agitate her with your complaints." I said that we shouldn't waste time as the contractions were already very intense. Nevertheless, I could not get rid of the husband, he was so adamant.

I opened the door of the delivery room and led the young woman in. I was about to close the door but the husband stopped me. I became frustrated. The mother's wailing intensified gradually and we were wasting our time with the husband. I forcefully demanded that he go home, since he couldn't be present at the delivery. When he said no, I asked him at least to let me examine his wife in private so that I could roughly predict the time of delivery. He conceded this, but he said he would sit at the door and would not leave until I let him in. He had promised not to leave his wife's side ever and he would keep this promise. He thus sat on the doorstep.

I could finally examine the woman. It was her first delivery, and she was in the cervical dilation phase. I told the man that he could go home because the delivery would not take place until morning. I was reassuring him, saying that his wife was in good hands and he could come to see the results by morning. He couldn't sit on the doorstep all night after all.

It seemed pointless to tell him anything at this point. When I closed the door, he ran outside to the room's window and asked his wife to come out because he wanted to see her just for a moment.

I noticed that this fuss had started to bother the woman as well, who was in great pain and needed peace. The woman told me that her husband's love was tiresome to her too, but what was to be done when her husband had such intense feelings towards her? While the man was shouting from the window, I locked the door and went back to the patient. I assumed he would change his mind outside in the cold and would go home sooner or later.

A nice, healthy boy was born by two in the morning. I took care of both of them; and when I saw that they looked all right and the mother fell asleep, I went to bed too.

In the morning we were woken up by an intense pounding on the door. It was the husband there before sunrise to see if his wife had survived the delivery. I told him that she had. In fact, she survived it with a healthy, newborn baby boy. Nonetheless, his wife was exhausted and fell asleep not long ago; so we should leave her in peace, I added. He said he would stay there as long as it took to see his wife. I realized that I could not get rid of him easily so I let him take a look at his wife from the doorstep. However, I asked him kindly not to enter the room.

I expected him to calm down upon seeing his wife sleeping nicely in bed and witnessing that everything was all right.

And yet this expectation turned out to be too optimistic. He approached the door quietly on his toes; and when I opened it a bit, he thrust it wide open with a sudden move and stormed into the room. He ran to his wife, clung to her, shook her up, kissed her and announced that no one would remove him from this bed not even by force.

With great effort I managed to make him leave the room, which was more exhausting than the delivery itself. I was counting the days and looking forward to seeing the end of the eight-day period when we could finally let the mother go home. The annoyance we had to go through with this man in the meantime was unbelievable.

This mother showed up fourteen months later at our clinic and, probably due to the hands of providence, I was the one who happened to be on duty again. I recognized her in an instant. I saw that she was about to have a delivery. I looked around in a gaze of terror, expecting to see her infamous husband turn up. I became frightened that this man's passionate love might complicate things again.

The woman shamefully lowered her head to the ground and whispered that she came alone this time. "Alone?" I asked with astonishment. "How come? Perhaps your husband is working and is unaware that the delivery is about to take place?" "Oh no," she replied. "My husband has left me. We've got divorced."

"That's impossible! He was so passionate about you. What actually happened?" I asked. "Well, we didn't see eye to eye when we returned home from the clinic. Our baby completely changed our life. Things never went back to normal. My husband wanted me to spend all my time with him instead of with the baby. Then, he abruptly left me," she replied.

I couldn't imagine how this poor woman would make a living and take care of her two babies on her own. She told me that her grandmother would babysit them while she tried to find work somewhere. From the money she could earn, they would try to get by somehow.

Eventually she gave birth to a nice girl by the morning. Nevertheless, this poor woman remained very sad. Nobody stormed into the room this time, and there was no man who said how much he loved her and would never leave her side.

I tried to console her by saying that her ex-husband would definitely come back to her if he found out about this beautiful baby girl. "That'll be the day," she said. "It was exactly when he heard that another baby was on the way that he decided to leave. Besides, it is rumored that he is courting some other woman and plans to get married again."

The woman was right; her husband didn't come to see her even once. It seemed he wasn't even interested in the children. As he was not helping them financially either, the grandmother helped the mother bring up the little ones while the young woman worked tirelessly to make ends meet.

And hence, this was how the husband's passionate love ended. The husband didn't keep his promise not to ever leave her wife's side even for a moment. In fact, it was ultimately not only his wife's side that he abandoned but also that of his children.

WAR DOES NOT STOP DELIVERIES

The Soviet Union launched an operation in 1944 to push Nazi-German troops out of Hungary. Fighting was already intense close to our village as Soviet troops quickly advanced into the country, but the Germans, nevertheless, still held out here and there.

As for women, they delivered during the war too; and as for me, I was called to deliveries no matter the sound of guns and artillery. A young boy ran to my place, saying that his mother didn't feel well and asked me to see her. His father wasn't home; he had been taken to forced labor.

I took the boy's hand and we left with him leading the way. We were trying to use the buildings as cover from the artillery. They were shooting nonstop but we couldn't figure out which direction it came from. It was reassuring that nothing was hit near us and no buildings were damaged. "This could mean that the line of combat is still a good distance from us," I thought to myself. We didn't see soldiers either, so we crossed each street with more and more confidence.

I found the patient with another small child at home. She was already in an advanced phase of her delivery and sighed in an air of relief when she saw me. As the delivery progressed nicely, we kept hearing the artillery fire gradually getting closer. I tried to figure out where I could take this woman for safety. I was afraid too, of course; but I, unlike other people, could not run to the public shelter at this moment. I sent the two children to the kitchen to boil some water for the baby's upcoming bathing. At least, I thought, they would be busy and wouldn't be in the way.

An hour later, a nice, healthy boy was born without any complications. As I was taking care of the patient and bathing her baby, a man ran into the room. He said he received word that a woman had had her delivery performed here. They were already asking everyone to find some shelter from the upcoming battle and we should do so as well.

I became frightened since I didn't know how and where I could take this woman. If we lifted and moved her right after delivery that could cause excessive bleeding and there was no doctor nearby.

The man turned out to be extremely helpful. He said he had heard about a large house a few streets down with a spacious cellar that had been turned into a shelter. We could take the woman there with his help. He ran home to fetch a wheelbarrow. I put pillows in it and placed the mother inside, covered with blankets. The man started to cautiously push the wheelbarrow so as not to shake the mother too hard. I led the two children with one hand and held the newborn in the other.

Unfortunately, by the time we reached the cellar, it was already occupied by four families. They did not want to let us in as the place was already overcrowded beyond its capacity. Nevertheless, our man was quite capable and didn't give in. He kept pushing the cellar's door that was kept shut by the people inside and explained that this woman had just given birth to a child and had two other children with her and therefore could not be left outside. Eventually, they pitied us and let us in. One of the families even offered a thick eiderdown that the mother could use to lie down on. The two children and I sat down around her.

I kept an eye on the mother to see if she started to bleed in this turmoil. The road, apparently, had not distressed her and everything seemed all right.

We kept anxiously silent as we were listening to the alternately sharpening and fading sound of the artillery. We arrived at the shelter in the morning; and before we noticed, the day had slowly turned into late afternoon. Needless to say, nobody had brought food to the shelter, as they expected to be hiding there only for a couple of hours. Thus, the children started to become hungry.

One of them started to complain out loud. Chaos broke out and every child started to beg for food unanimously as a large choir. The mother had also got hungry in the meantime and said she could not put up with this starving. She felt for her children too. She said she had recovered her strength and would go home to fetch some food.

At her announcement, someone commented that the troops must have advanced beyond our area because no firing had been heard for a long time. It really was quiet as we listened. We cautiously opened the shelter's iron door and peeked out; the streets were completely empty. We couldn't imagine what had happened, but the whole area was in perfect silence indeed.

Considering that the mother couldn't move right after delivery and given the unusual state of peace, I asked her where I could find food at her house. She said that she was craving some chicken soup at that moment. She lent me her oldest child to help me. She said that I would find ingredients for the soup in the pantry, provided that the firefight was truly over and I had the courage to prepare it.

The other child was hungry as well, so I left with both of them to fetch some food. The fact that we didn't hear shots fired on the way encouraged us a little. The children found some bread to eat at home and spread lard on it. I prepared two chickens and put them in a large bowl with plenty of vegetables to cook. I thought that this soup would satisfy the mother even without the chicken meat properly cooked in it.

I put all the food I could find in a basket while the soup was cooking. The meat was cooking nicely too when, all of a sudden, shots were fired again. This time they sounded close to us.

I looked outside the window and saw that the next house's chimney had just been shot down. I quickly took the bowl, covered it and placed it in another basket. I took the two baskets and left with the children. The way back was not as easy as our way to the house had been. The air was full of dust either in front of or behind us. The fire and return fire started to intensify. The two children took cover trembling behind my back.

Moving from cover to cover, from one house to the next, we eventually reached the shelter with the two baskets. They had locked the iron door of the cellar fearing that shrapnel might fly inside or an enemy soldier might find his way in.

We knocked and banged on the door and shouted to get them to open it, but it was all in vain—the door didn't move. As we later learned, they had only noticed the banging on the door but did not hear our voices; therefore, they wouldn't let anyone in, fearing that enemy soldiers were trying to get inside. The children and I desperately took shelter at the bottom of the door during the greatest artillery fire. The kids started to cry in fear.

After a long time, as the gunfire had ceased, we started to bang on the door again. Inside, the poor, weak mother, who had suspected that it was us the first time too, begged the people to open the door, but they resisted her.

Now that silence had returned, they opened the door a bit to peek out. When they saw us, they were relieved and we were quickly let in. I fed the mother who was revitalized by the soup. The children ate again and we shared the remaining soup equally among the people present.

Someone decided to peek out of the door again. He said he might have seen an enemy soldier running past the neighboring house. A couple of people from the shelter ventured out and saw Soviet soldiers drawing pieces of artillery with horses. When the soldiers noticed us in the cellar door, they waved and gestured that there was nothing to fear and we could come out since the battle was over. Nobody dared to leave the shelter at this point, of course.

It was late at night when Soviet soldiers knocked on the cellar door and gestured again that we could go home because all the Germans were gone. They also noticed the newborn. They picked him up, cuddled and caressed him telling each other how cute the newborn was. After this event we were a bit relieved and started to think about preparing to go back to our abandoned homes.

Despite all this fighting, the Germans did make a comeback later on.

REFUGE AT THE CLINIC

After a few days' pause, the battle started all over. This time the Germans occupied the village and warned the local population to leave their homes and flee. Many feared a large battle would occur around the town and moved to distant farms, to relatives or to friends. The officials of the village also left among many others. Because I had neither relatives nor friends who could provide me with shelter, I thought I would move into the obstetrical clinic and take refuge there until the fighting ended. At the same time, I would guard the equipment and devices so that they wouldn't get stolen during the chaos.

I was completely alone at the clinic. The janitor who normally came at noon had also fled the village. There was a huge turmoil in the settlement; soldiers urged everyone to leave their homes. They apparently forgot about me, as no one bothered to warn anyone at the clinic. It seems they couldn't imagine anybody could be staying there.

I was starting to hear the artillery fire when a carriage stopped in front of the entrance. It brought a pregnant mother from a farm. The mother still felt well enough and came inside on her own while her husband was taking care of the horses. I examined the mother and asked if she had seen a doctor previously, because I felt she had a narrow pelvic bone. Yes, she had seen a doctor who told her exactly the same and said that she could only deliver her baby in a hospital because of her physical condition. The doctor had previously told the couple that this would not be a straightforward delivery. This is why they had come to the clinic; they were terrified that the delivery might start on their way here.

I waited until her husband came in and explained to the two of them that this was only a small country clinic and not a hospital. No operations could be carried out here, especially not when military combat was taking place near the village. I couldn't even call a doctor here at that point, because everybody had left the place and I was staying here on my own. Without a doctor, however, I could not perform this delivery. Still, they had come using a carriage, so I advised the woman's husband to take his wife to the city hospital as her contractions were not yet intense and they might have enough time to act and possibly make it to the city.

The woman understood my words right away. It seems she had been well-informed about her case by her doctor and was about to go back to the carriage, but her husband was unwilling to leave. He started complaining aloud that I only wanted to get rid of them because I was scared and wanted to flee at once. He announced they would stay at the clinic.

I drew the husband aside and told him that this would foreseeably be a very complicated delivery and both the baby's and the mother's lives might be on the line. I would be unable to save his wife on my own in case of an emergency, and there was no doctor nearby to help us. This quieted him down a bit, but hardly had I finished my monologue before a massive artillery fire hit close by and was followed by others. The three of us hurried into the delivery room in horror.

Well, that settled it, the man said. He trusted me to help his wife with my greatest knowledge. There was no way to go into the hospital from this point on, as shots were fired from every direction. I had to admit that the situation was hopeless and I felt for the mother. It was still preferable for her to stay at the clinic than to have her delivery in the carriage in the midst of the lines of fire.

I asked the man to move the carriage and tie the horses in a safe place where the animals wouldn't flee in case they got scared by the noise and then to come back and sit in the clinic's corridor because I would be needing his help. However, he didn't mean to stay at the clinic himself. Instead, he wanted to leave the village to go back to his farm. He didn't want to leave the farm deserted when the soldiers arrived and he had plenty of cattle to feed anyway.

It was absolutely unacceptable to see the only person who could help me leave. I asked him what was more important: the life of his wife and the baby or the farm with the cattle? The thought that I would be left alone with this poor woman in this foreseeably complicated delivery frightened me. I had no chance to find anyone else in the village whom I could count on except the husband. When I was laying the woman on the bed, her husband quietly sneaked out of the room. By the time I realized his absence, he had whipped the horses and quickly ridden away. He didn't even say goodbye to his wife so as not to risk being kept there by her!

What are we going to do now? I thought to myself. I didn't want to upset the mother because her pain was intensifying and the target location of the artillery fire was approaching us fast. I prepared everything for the delivery and ran to the telephone to call some prominent members in the village. I tried calling the doctor's house several times, but it was all in vain since nobody answered.

The situation was completely hopeless; everybody had left the village. I decided to stop trying to reach people on the phone and instead disinfected my hands and examined the mother again. I expected a painful delivery for her. The head of the fetus did not fit in the aperture of the pelvis at all but rather was positioned in a way that evaded the entrance of the womb. In a hospital they would definitely have performed a Caesarian section. Only a miracle could help us and the calm behavior of the woman.

She was a smart, quick-witted young wife. During a pause between two contractions I explained to her that the delivery's outcome ultimately depended on her behavior. I told her exactly what to do in certain instances. I could tell that she realized that from that point on only the two of us were fighting for her life, without any external assistance. I prepared her for the possibility that the baby might not make it alive, but we would do everything to save at least her own life. "Just listen carefully and patiently to my advice and do as I say, and eventually it will be fine," I tried to calm her in a rather uncertain tone.

The contractions intensified and hours passed by, but the delivery did not seem to progress. Although the artillery fire got even closer, we were concentrating so hard that we scarcely noticed it. The cervix had dilated but the fetus's head could still not fit in the aperture of the pelvis, and, of course, there was neither a doctor nor an injection in sight to help us. Even though we were not allowed to give injections as midwives, I was ready to give one at that point had we had one in the clinic. Unfortunately, we were forbidden to keep either injections or medicine there. They were always brought in by the doctors themselves.

I kept thinking about how I could fit the fetus's head in the aperture. I took a blanket and wrapped it around the mother's body and used the clothing between two contractions to push the fetus' head in the right direction. Then, I pulled the blanket and tied it tightly so as to keep the head still and not to let it go back into its initial position during the next contraction.

When I was done with it, I told the patient to hold the bed railing and push with all her strength during the next contraction.

We struggled with this method for hours and we both became exhausted without any success. This poor woman, nevertheless, listened carefully to my advice and wanted to help, but the labor did not progress. I listened to the fetus's heartbeat, which was still satisfying at the time. The thought that we might save the fetus encouraged me. Both of my hands were numb from the constant pushing, when I suddenly noticed that the fetus' head had moved into the aperture.

This doubled our determination. We didn't even hear the artillery anymore; we had enough troubles at the moment and sweat was literally pouring off us.

We were struggling for eight hours until we became completely exhausted. We had to power through this period under primitive conditions until the mother's baby was born. He was a boy; but after all the pressure of this delivery, he was born with algid asphyxia, meaning that both the baby's respiration and circulation were unsatisfactory. Nevertheless, the heartbeat was still promising. I saw that the mother was relieved after the events and asked right away whether the baby made it.

I said I still heard heartbeats and I would do everything I could to save the baby's life. The mother was not bleeding, so I put a blanket over her and quickly started to revive the baby. Although my hands and feet were trembling from exhaustion and I was afraid of dropping the baby, taking a break was out of the question at the time.

I extracted saliva, and gave a hot-cold bath to the baby, but he didn't react. Then, I tried swaying him: lifting his head down in order to make the chest constrict and then turning him around to induce the air to flow into his lungs. I repeated this several times and then used the hot-cold bath again, but he gave no signs of life, even though his heartbeats were still satisfactory. "I've got to hold out, I can't give it up now," I tried to encourage myself.

For two hours I tried everything I had ever learned or read about reviving moribund babies, when the baby finally turned blue. I felt hope again. More hot-cold baths, swaying and slapping followed until the baby finally cried out loud. I have never heard such a beautiful cry since! We both shed tears of joy. We forgot altogether our anguish that we had suffered for roughly one and a half days up to that point. The suffering was given meaning all at once.

I quickly covered the baby with clothing and hurried back to the mother to take a look at her, because while I was taking care of the baby, I couldn't even deal with the mother, only kept asking her whether she was all right, was she bleeding and so on. When I finally had the chance to examine the mother again, I couldn't believe my eyes. After all this torment she didn't even have a simple perineal tear! She was all right apart from the normal signs of the event.

I bathed the baby, swaddled him and put him in a crib that I pulled close to the mother. Then, I brought an extra bed in the room for myself. I locked the door and the three of us fell asleep in no time, as if we weren't in the middle of the war within deadly artillery fire all around us.

I woke up to people pounding on the door. I got up, put on a cloak and, though being somewhat afraid myself, opened the door an inch. Soviet soldiers were standing in the corridor. I let them into the delivery room where we were staying with the mother and, since I didn't speak their language, tried to gesture to them somehow that this was an obstetrical clinic and showed them the newborn. Many others came in and finally a translator showed up who said they hadn't found anyone in the village apart from us and a couple of people hiding in cellars. In fact, they didn't expect to find anyone at the clinic at all. They explained that since the inhabitants had fled the area, foreseeably there wouldn't be deliveries at the clinic for a while and instead it would be turned into a hospital. Of course, they let us stay there to wait for the mother's husband to pick her up.

Three days after this event the husband showed up at the clinic and was nervous to find out whether her wife had survived the delivery or not. To his immense surprise, he found both his wife and the newborn alive at the clinic.

The woman didn't even develop a fever, so I put blankets in her husband's carriage for her to sit on, gave advice to the young couple concerning their baby and saw them off.

When life returned to normal, they came back along with the baby to visit me. He was an exceptionally vivid, adorable little boy frolicking in his swaddling clothes. I couldn't believe my eyes! Was he really the baby who needed so many hours to be brought back to life?

Later on, we kept saying together with the mother that perhaps no one else apart from the three of us in the whole country could boast to have endured the Soviet advance fast asleep in bed.

MIDWIFE AT THE CLINIC

After Hungary's Soviet occupation, I continued my profession as a private midwife. Since there was now an obstetrical clinic in our village, no more community midwives were appointed by the state in the area. At the clinic, they still tried to provide staff by asking midwives to be on duty on a scheduled basis.

The objective of the village was to encourage women to have their deliveries at the clinic. To this end, they extended their capacity, furnished new rooms, increased the number of beds, acquired modern equipment and provided excellent service for the mothers. Despite all these efforts, the women still felt a distrust of delivering at the clinic. In spite of the fact that doctors and the village officials made huge efforts to persuade women to visit the clinic, everybody wanted to deliver at home, so, to a certain point, this effort remained all in vain.

In the meantime, news of me starting my private practice again spread all over the village, and I was asked for from one delivery to another. Whereas my share of deliveries was ten to fifteen a month in my private practice, only one or two were performed at the clinic. Needless to say, I tried to persuade the mothers with great effort to visit the clinic, because it was hard for a person my age to perform so many deliveries on a regular basis and check up on the mothers during the following eight days.

On one exceptionally cold, snowy day, I arrived home from my second delivery. It was late in the afternoon and I was so tired I didn't even have the strength to kindle the stove, so I went to sleep in the ice-cold room. Because of the cold and exhaustion, however, I couldn't fall asleep. Suddenly, somebody knocked on my door. I thought I wouldn't answer to give them the impression that no one was at home and thus make them take the mother to the clinic. Nevertheless, this person kept on knocking persistently. I couldn't bear it anymore and got up to ask who it was.

"Oh, it is such a relief to find you at home," a man said. "Please come with me quickly because contractions have started with my wife." "Unfortunately, I cannot go with you now," I answered. "I have already performed two deliveries today and I am afraid of making a mistake due to my tiredness. But the obstetrical clinic should be open, so you can take your wife there." "My wife would never agree to that," he replied. "She insists on seeing Miss Mária. But please come quickly as she is feeling very bad already!"

Eventually, I couldn't say no. As usual, I got dressed quickly, as I always do so as not to endanger the mothers' lives by taking my time. The man came with a carriage and told me not to worry because he had brought warm sheepskin clothing so I wouldn't be cold on the way. We headed out to his farm.

Given the circumstances of the day I was not surprised that the delivery was accompanied with complications—the fetus was lying in a transverse position in the womb. Normally, we would need a doctor for this sort of delivery but that could mean hours of travelling in a carriage for the doctor. Given the situation I was facing the usual challenges of my profession on my own. In the end, as happened in most of the cases, I managed to perform the delivery without any major problems.

I arrived home once again, but this time I kindled the stove because the room was so cold I knew I definitely couldn't fall asleep at that temperature. I got used to not checking the time when I went to bed. I didn't sleep when everyone else usually did, but rather as soon as I got home from work. The room got nicely warmed up and I was getting ready to go to bed when I noticed someone knocking on my door again. I looked outside and saw the judge of the local court standing there. He asked me to let him in; he wanted to discuss something with me.

I presumed he hadn't come here concerning a delivery as he was on the wrong side of fifty. Other than that, I had no idea what he wanted to discuss with me, as I was no longer a community midwife.

"It was decided," the judge started his speech, "that the local doctor and I should formally ask if you could undertake the management of the area's obstetrical clinic, and to this end move there? The position comes with an apartment near the place at your disposal so that the clinic can have a permanent midwife. I believe, Miss Mária, that we share the same goal: to persuade the local women to have their deliveries at the clinic. Our village has spent a great deal of money on this clinic and its capacity is still unused, regardless of the large number of deliveries taking place in the district. We know that expecting mothers love you very much and ask for you with great confidence. This is why our choice fell on you. If word spreads that you are running the clinic, people will flood there." I was a bit surprised by the judge's speech, to be honest. I said I couldn't give an answer at that point because I wanted to consult with the local doctor first.

The Chief Medical Officer of the region also encouraged me to accept the position because he thought this would help both the mothers and me. I could see the mothers in the clinic in sterile, healthy and humane conditions and with the available presence of a doctor on a permanent basis. And as for me, I could work more easily in a well-equipped workplace with a telephone to call a special doctor at any time in case of an emergency.

This argument struck a chord. They would provide me with a telephone and a doctor. I wouldn't have to visit distant farms anymore because the women would be brought to the clinic. I accepted the offer.

Before I moved into the clinic, I visited the expecting mothers one-by-one and told them to expect to have their deliveries at the clinic in case they wanted to have it performed by me. I said that as of the first day of the month, they couldn't ask for me, as I would be working at the clinic full-time.

And the mothers indeed visited the clinic after that. So many of them came that we were afraid of running out of our extended capacity. Whenever the Chief Medical Officer received official guests, he took them there and proudly showed them the highly-utilized clinic of the village.

FOOTNOTES

---

[1] The third largest city of Hungary and the center of the southern part of the Great Hungarian Plain.

[2] Pengő was the currency of Hungary between January 1, 1927 and July 31, 1946.

[3] A horsecar is a horse-drawn streetcar that runs on rails.

[4] In Hungarian, *gonosz szem* means "evil eye," but more widespread is the expression *szemmelverés* (lit. "beating with eye"), which refers to the alleged act of harming one by an evil look.

MIDWIFE'S EPILOGUE

In our modern society the role of midwives has been taken over by professional obstetricians, but in the old days I was practicing as a midwife, aiding and assisting the expecting mothers in the rural districts of the Great Hungarian Plain.

A midwife, according to one Hungarian Lexicon, is "a wicked spinster; the name is synonymous with a witch." An obstetrician, on the other hand—according to the same Lexicon—is "a person who is in charge of professionally taking care of and examining pregnant women and their newborns." We were midwives in the old days, but we were certainly not "wicked spinsters" or "witches." We were respected and loved by the community, and its members warmly called us "Auntie Midwives," or familiarly "Miss Mária" in my case. Not only did we take care of the examination of pregnant women, but we also performed deliveries with heroic bravery, under adverse conditions at lonely farms, far away from any doctor or inhabited place. We often strived on our own to save lives.

Nowadays, it seems incredible to me how I managed to practice this profession throughout a lifetime. I don't refer solely to the many nights that I spent in tension at the side of expecting mothers, hoping to save their lives and, if necessary, to send for a doctor on time, but also to the thought, for instance, that it never came to my mind to be afraid on the road.

On many occasions, nobody came to me directly from the mother's family; instead, they sent a messenger to let me know where my help was needed. I left on foot no matter how dark it was outside or how abandoned I felt on the way. If my road happened to lead through a cemetery, I crossed it even at midnight. I was never afraid, I only tried to hurry so as not to be late!

Often, strangers came to my place and asked me to go with them. It never crossed my mind that they might not even be taking me to a delivery but were instead planning on robbing me on the way. My only concern was to arrive to the delivery on time.

I was not afraid on country roads, or in the cemetery, or in the dark. I was afraid of neither people nor unchained dogs. It is also noteworthy to mention that my trust in the world never let me down. No one ever hurt me during my career.

Though the above-mentioned quote from the Lexicon made me smile from time to time, I knew that we, as midwives, were perceived neither as "spinsters" nor as "witches" by our community. The truth was simpler and more prosaic than that: People always loved and respected their local midwife.

APPENDIX

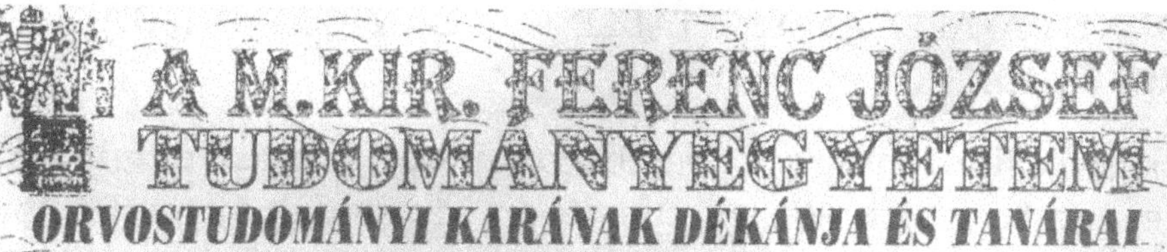

English translation of the Original Degree

18/1928. O.K.sz.

WE

THE DEAN AND PROFESSORS OF THE MEDICAL FACULTY OF THE ROYAL HUNGARIAN FRANZ JOSEPH UNIVERSITY

Certify and announce it to anyone whom it may concern that reputable MÁRIA SZÉCSI (wife of András Nemes), who was born in Simonyifalva in the year 1900, received regular theoretical and practical instruction in 1927-28 by the Midwifery Institution of the Gynecologist Clinic of the Royal Hungarian Franz Joseph University, underwent strict examination in our presence concerning her knowledge on the below-mentioned date, gave thorough proof of her practical expertise and thus she WAS FOUND CAPABLE AND SUITABLE TO PRACTICE THE MIDWIFERY PROFESSION.

On the basis of these criteria, the graduate having solemnly taken the statutory oath, WE, by the power invested in us by the Royal Hungarian Ministry and under her unconditional observation of the solemnly sworn oath and provided her precise compliance with the bonding instructions and regulations thereof, accept Mária Szécsi (wife of András Nemes) as a qualified and competent midwife and HEREBY AUTHORIZE HER TO THE OPEN PRACTICE OF MIDWIFERY.

To this end, the Royal Hungarian Franz Joseph University—certified with its own seal and confirmed by the present professors' genuine signatures—issued a

DEGREE

to the aforementioned graduate's disposal.

Issued in Szeged, June 21, 1928

Dr. József Szabó   Dr. János Berecz
Tenured Professor   Tenured Professor
Annual Dean of the Medical Faculty   Principal of the Gynecologist Clinic

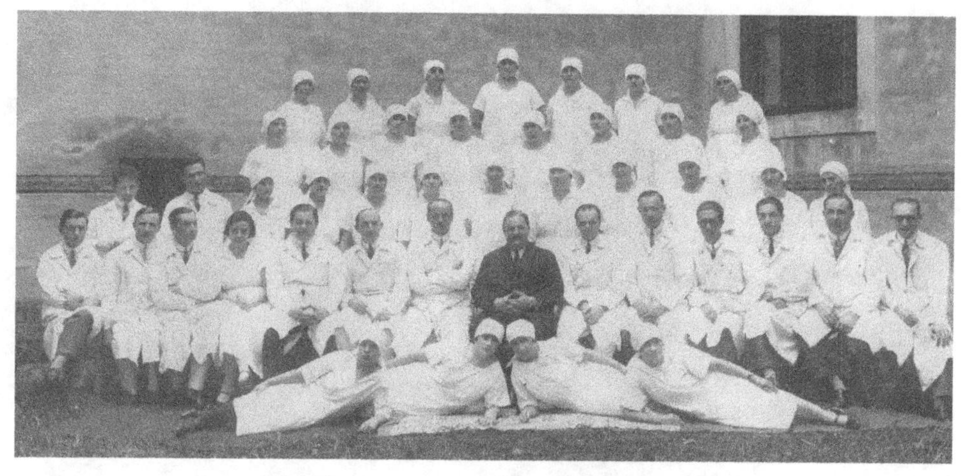

Graduating class of the 1927-28 midwifery program at Szeged

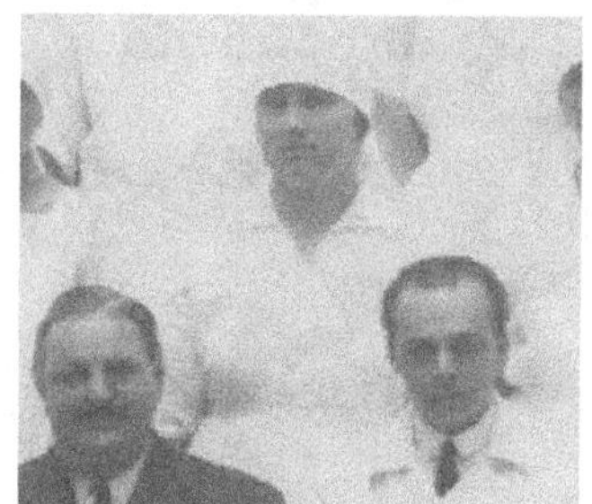

Close-up of Mária Szécsi

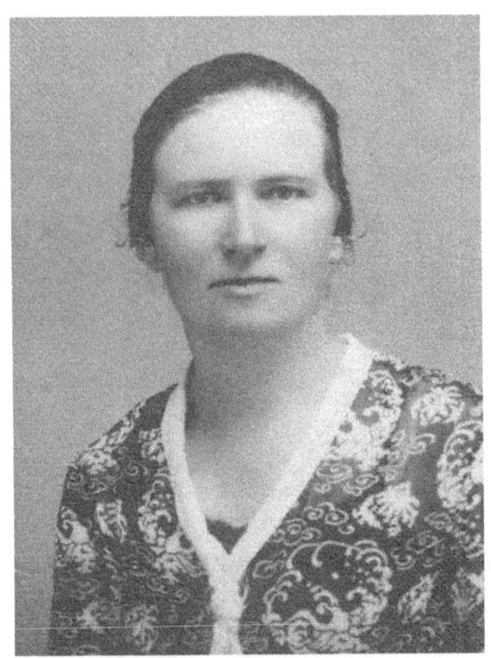

"Auntie Midwife"

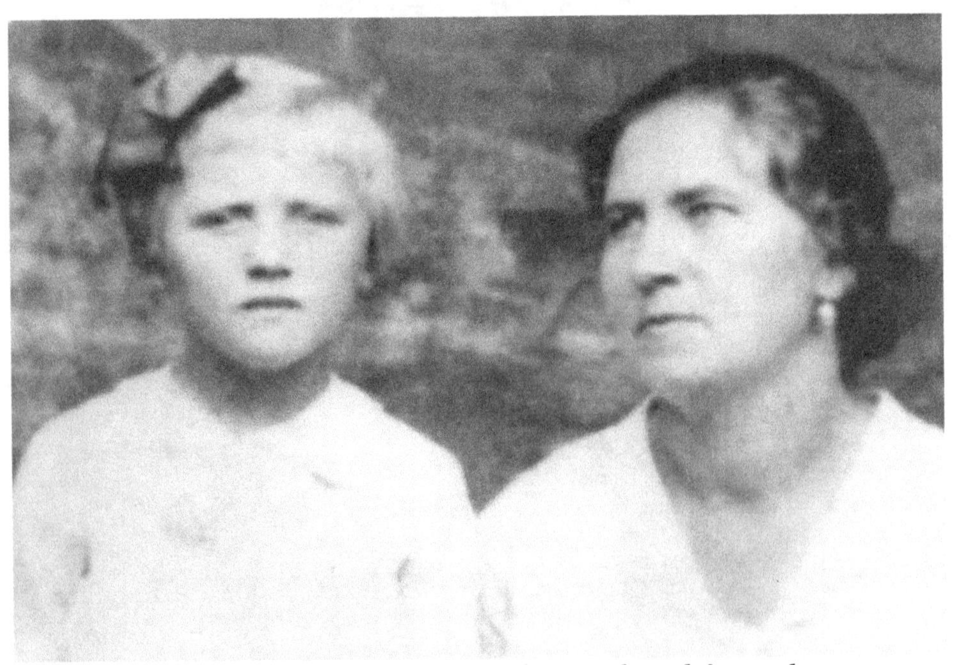

Mária Szécsi with her daughter, who ultimately
inspired the publication of this book